Understanding Intelligence

Have you ever wondered why psychologists still can't agree on what intelligence is? Or felt dismayed by debates around individual differences? Criticising the pitfalls of IQ testing, this book explains the true nature of intelligent systems, and their evolution from cells to brains to culture and human minds.

Understanding Intelligence debunks many of the myths and misunderstandings surrounding intelligence. It takes a new look at the nature of the environment and the development of 'talent' and achievement. This brings fresh and radical implications for promoting intelligence and creativity, and prompts readers to reconsider their own possibilities and aspirations.

Providing a broad context to the subject, the author also unmasks the ideological distortions of intelligence in racism and eugenics, and the suppressed expectations across social classes and genders.

This book is a must-read for anyone curious about our own intelligence.

Ken Richardson is a former senior lecturer at the Open University, UK, and an independent researcher, consultant, and author. After completing a doctorate in brain biochemistry he became interested in cognitive systems, chiefly developmental, and how these areas, as intelligent systems, are inter-related through evolution.

The **Understanding Life** series is for anyone wanting an engaging and concise way into a key biological topic. Offering a multidisciplinary perspective, these accessible guides address common misconceptions and misunderstandings in a thoughtful way to help stimulate debate and encourage a more in-depth understanding. Written by leading thinkers in each field, these books are for anyone wanting an expert overview that will enable clearer thinking on each topic.

Series Editor: Kostas Kampourakis http://kampourakis.com

Published titles

Understanding Evolution	Kostas Kampourakis	9781108746083
Understanding Coronavirus	Raul Rabadan	9781108826716
Understanding Development	Alessandro Minelli	9781108799232
Understanding Evo-Devo	Wallace Arthur	9781108819466
Understanding Genes	Kostas Kampourakis	9781108812825
Understanding DNA Ancestry	Sheldon Krimsky	9781108816038
Understanding Intelligence	Ken Richardson	9781108940368
Understanding Metaphors in the Life Sciences	Andrew S. Reynolds	9781108940498

Forthcoming

Understanding Creationism	Glenn Branch	9781108927505
Understanding Species	John S. Wilkins	9781108987196
Understanding the Nature–Nurture Debate	Eric Turkheimer	9781108958165
Understanding How Science Explains the World	Kevin McCain	9781108995504
Understanding Cancer	Robin Hesketh	9781009005999
Understanding Forensic DNA	Suzanne Bell and John Butler	9781009044011
Understanding Race	Rob DeSalle and Ian Tattersall	9781009055581
Understanding Fertility	Gab Kovacs	9781009054164

Understanding Intelligence

KEN RICHARDSON
Formerly of the Open University, UK

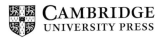

CAMBRIDGE
UNIVERSITY PRESS

CAMBRIDGE
UNIVERSITY PRESS

University Printing House, Cambridge CB2 8BS, United Kingdom

One Liberty Plaza, 20th Floor, New York, NY 10006, USA

477 Williamstown Road, Port Melbourne, VIC 3207, Australia

314–321, 3rd Floor, Plot 3, Splendor Forum, Jasola District Centre,
New Delhi – 110025, India

103 Penang Road, #05–06/07, Visioncrest Commercial, Singapore 238467

Cambridge University Press is part of the University of Cambridge.

It furthers the University's mission by disseminating knowledge in the pursuit of
education, learning, and research at the highest international levels of excellence.

www.cambridge.org
Information on this title: www.cambridge.org/9781108837132
DOI: 10.1017/9781108937757

First published 2022

Printed in the United Kingdom by TJ Books Limited, Padstow Cornwall

A catalogue record for this publication is available from the British Library.

Library of Congress Cataloging-in-Publication Data
Names: Richardson, Ken, author.
Title: Understanding intelligence / Ken Richardson, Formerly of the Open University, UK.
Description: 1 Edition. | r, New York, NY : Cambridge University Press, 2021. | Series:
Understanding life | Includes index.
Identifiers: LCCN 2021022821 (print) | LCCN 2021022822 (ebook) | ISBN 9781108837132
(hardback) | ISBN 9781108940368 (paperback) | ISBN 9781108937757 (ebook)
Subjects: LCSH: Eugenics. | Intellect. | Intelligence levels. | BISAC: MEDICAL / Neuroscience
Classification: LCC HQ751 .R53 2021 (print) | LCC HQ751 (ebook) | DDC 363.9/2–dc23
LC record available at https://lccn.loc.gov/2021022821
LC ebook record available at https://lccn.loc.gov/2021022822

ISBN 978-1-108-83713-2 Hardback
ISBN 978-1-108-94036-8 Paperback

'Ken Richardson has written a masterful book about intelligence. In contrast to what leading behavioural geneticists and psychometrically oriented psychologists see as the moderately or highly heritable trait of general intelligence (IQ), Richardson explains why psychometric and behavioural genetic arguments fail, and how intelligence should be seen as a socially acquired characteristic. A longstanding expert on intelligence, he writes in a manner that can be understood by both academic and general readers. I strongly recommend this book as an accessible and important counterweight to mainstream descriptions of intelligence in the fields of psychology and behavioural genetics, and in the media.'
 Jay Joseph, Psy.D., psychologist and author, Oakland, California, USA

'Ken Richardson's *Understanding Intelligence* is a timely and important addition to Cambridge University Press's groundbreaking Understanding Life series. Richardson provides a "natural history of intelligence", and no facet of that complex topic goes untouched – adaptive evolution, embryology, endocrinology, circadian rhythms, neural networks, cooperative hunting. In our current moment, where scholars and politicians alike are calling for gene-guided education and appealing to innate differences as the cause of racial disparities, Richardson debunks myth after myth about cognitive ability: that the brain is best conceptualised as a machine, that IQ tests measure intelligence, that different racial groups have naturally different intellectual aptitudes, that the genome is a programme for cognitive development. The esteemed psychologist, in exchange, offers a vision of intelligence as a dynamic, interactive, developing, adaptive system – a system that allows every person to intellectually flourish, if only they are given the opportunity.'
        James Tabery, Professor of Philosophy, University of Utah, USA

'For decades, Ken Richardson has been a leading voice within the critical approaches to intelligence in psychology. He patiently and determinedly interrogated the often taken for granted assumptions – and myths – about the meaning of intelligence, about how it can be measured and tested, about its heritability or its applicability as a measure of intellectual ability in the school or the workplace. *Understanding Intelligence* provides a thoroughly researched and persuasively argued up-to-date overview of this important work. It is sure to become an indispensable resource for both academics and practitioners, and indeed for anyone interested in one of psychology's most controversial, and flawed, concepts.'
Jovan Byford, Senior Lecturer in Psychology, The Open University, UK

Contents

Foreword

What is intelligence? People often take the answer to this question as simple and straightforward. It seems to be about how 'smart' one is, and to be considered something that can be easily and objectively measured, for example, by how good at math one is, or by how well one does in problem-solving. There even exist smartphone apps that claim to measure one's intelligence. Or so the story goes. Intelligence is an attribute that is considered a good one, yet it is one of the most used ones to support discrimination. This was most prominently shown during the era of eugenics, when people described as 'feebleminded' might even be sterilised in order to be precluded from reproducing. But this is not over. Several prominent people nowadays still argue about the intellectual superiority of men over women; of 'white' people over 'black' people; of humans over other species. This is based on an important assumption: that we can accurately and unbiasedly measure intelligence. In this magnificent book Ken Richardson shows that it is far from simple and straightforward not only to measure intelligence, but also to define it. The author explains the biases of the widely known IQ tests, and their validity problems. Most importantly, he advances a broader conceptualisation of intelligence that will make you realise that it is a lot more than the narrow set of skills measured by IQ tests. It is a property of life, one that we should admire and not use for discrimination. To paraphrase a famous saying: several decades of unwarranted discrimination are enough.

Kostas Kampourakis, Series Editor

Preface

Superficially, intelligence seems so easy to understand. It's what most separates us from all other animals; as defining of humanity as flying is of birds or swimming is of fish. It's also one of the first things we note in distinguishing people from one another. You may mention to friends that so-and-so is 'intelligent', perhaps using a common word such as 'smart' or 'bright'. They will tend to nod as if we all know what we mean.

What we really mean will usually be rather vague, though. In spite of a constant presence in our lives and institutions, it comes with variable connotations. What we mean divides left and right in politics; legitimises people's places on social ladders; raises daunting issues about equality and social justice; and has long been used to justify different treatments of genders, social classes, and 'races', as well as some appalling acts done in the name of this concept.

How are we to understand it then? What is it, really? Scholars, from Ancient Greece to modern times, have wrestled with that question. Today, psychologists often think they've cracked it by presenting us with 'definitions' of intelligence. Take the recent example of Richard Haier (author of *The Neuroscience of Intelligence*, 2016) and Stuart Ritchie (author of *Intelligence: All that Matters*, 2018). Both adopt Linda Gottfredson's definition (from an article in 1997):

> [Intelligence] ... involves the ability to reason, plan, solve problems, think abstractly, comprehend complex ideas, learn quickly and learn from experience. It is not merely book learning, a narrow academic skill,

or test-taking smarts. Rather it reflects a broader and deeper capability for comprehending our surroundings – 'catching on', 'making sense' of things, or 'figuring out' what to do.

I hope you've got that – 'catching on', 'making sense', or 'figuring out' are hardly pristine scientific concepts. Nor (as we shall see) is there a lot of agreement about the real nature of reasoning, problem-solving, and so on. The problem is that definitions only sketch the *boundaries* of a function; outlining what it does or does not do, without describing the function itself. Definitions *ad nauseam* do not tell us much about intelligent functions, how they originated, develop, and materialise in such splendid and variable forms. Telling us all the things that a machine or computer can do does not tell us how they do it.

So the old joke still stands: ask a dozen psychologists what intelligence is and you'll get a dozen different answers. There's also that other one suggesting that 'intelligence is what intelligence tests test'. When it comes to describing what individual differences are differences *in*, we get simple mechanical metaphors – energy, power, strength, speed, capacity, and efficiency are common. Others are sharp, smart, bright, dull, and so on – again, hardly scientific. We *still* need to know what kind of function intelligence really is: not just what it does, but how it does what it does. Until we achieve that, the whole subject slips and slides like a wayward bar of soap under the shower.

Anyone might have expected objective (dare I say intelligent?) scientists to have solved the problem by now. Why not? Well, intelligence is not a neutral subject like liver functions or the immune system, researched dispassionately. Cutting across and smearing our streams of inquiry are other potent forces. The concept of intelligence, after all, has a huge bearing on social and political issues: as a supposed resource for a nation's economy; for selecting the right people for the right education, training, and jobs; and for justifying the ordering of people on a social ladder, with different treatments, powers, and privileges. That has stirred long-standing nature–nurture debates not entirely conducive to objective science.

Science is, of course, often funded and harnessed for socially practical ends. But different hunches or beliefs about intelligence reflect fundamentally different preconceptions of human nature. That is why intelligence has often become an ideological football. That's a danger we should understand, because 'applied intelligence' can lead to dire consequences. Historically, IQ testing has been intertwined with eugenics movements, as well as proving the genetic inferiority of the working classes and different 'races'. Sad things have been said and done in its name.

Many scientists are currently fearful of a new wave of such things. Nightmarish elements of the designer baby industry were portrayed in the 1997 film *GATTACA* (see Kostas Kampourakis' discussion in *Understanding Genes*). In his blog in 2014, later UK government adviser Dominic Cummings wrote that, when a sufficient number of 'IQ genes' have been identified, then the state might consider subsidising suitable couples for selecting 'the egg that has the highest prediction for IQ'. Meanwhile, on the futility of intervention in what he sees as natural forces, Boris Johnson (now, in 2021, UK prime minister), was warning that, 'Whatever you may think of the value of IQ tests it is surely relevant to a conversation about equality that as many as 16% of our species have an IQ below 85 while about 2 per cent have an IQ above 130 . . . The harder you shake the pack the easier it will be for some cornflakes to get to the top' (Third Margaret Thatcher Lecture, 2013).

Like a gale on a homing pigeon, such ideological forces have continuously blown objective inquiry off course and onto troubled reefs. Yet, intelligence remains a subject of genuine scientific interest to many biologists, psychologists, philosophers, sociologists, and anthropologists. For generations, they have asked genuine questions: What is it? How did it originate? How did it evolve? What form does it take in humans and in individuals? How does it vary, both across species and between humans as individuals?

Meanwhile, results pouring out from other fields – biophysics, genetics, molecular biology, physiology, evolutionary studies, brain sciences, cognitive psychology, and others – have been spinning out new strands needing to be pulled together. They are beginning to cohere into a compelling story. It says that intelligence is not something only in our brains and, thanks to their genes, good in only Johnson's top 2 per cent. Rather, it has been at the very roots of life from the beginning, impelling evolution, emerging further in brains and cognitive systems, and re-emerging in unsuspected, and sadly understated, forms in all humans.

Using those strands to bring intelligence to life is the ambition of this book. I try to present a kind of natural history of intelligence. My underlying message is: 'Intelligence is life; life is intelligence.' My hope in writing this book is that it will bring a better understanding of life's most wonderful phenomenon, and also that it will encourage people to banish fatalism and pessimism about their own abilities, and more confidently *create* their potential for democratic engagement.

One of the most exciting aspects of efforts such as this is that of working with the ideas of many other people. Those who have unwittingly helped are too numerous to name here, but I hope they recognise my thanks in these pages. A number of friends and colleagues did, however, take the trouble to plough through most or all of the pages to offer suggestions and criticism. I would like to particularly thank Mike Jones, Jay Joseph, Stephen Block, Meg Brown, Philip Thompson, Susan Richardson, and Annie Watt. They were probably more helpful than they know. I'm also grateful to series editor Kostas Kampourakis for being exceedingly detailed and thorough in helping to shape up the drafts. I can only hope the result is a worthy reflection of all that wisdom.

1 Testing, Testing

When people consider intelligence, they will first tend to think of IQ, and scores that distinguish people, one from another. They will also tend to think of those scores as describing something as much part of individuals' make-up as faces and fingerprints. Today, a psychologist who uses IQ tests and attempts to prove score differences are caused by genetic differences will be described as an 'expert' on intelligence. That indicates how influential IQ testing has become, and how much it has become part of society's general conceptual furniture.

And yet, it's never sat comfortably among us. Everyone – including experts – will agree that, whatever intelligence is, it's bound to be complex, enigmatic, and difficult to describe: probably the most intricate function ever evolved. To this day, psychologists argue over what it actually is. So how has measuring it become so easy and apparently so convincing? Most IQ tests take around half an hour, though they vary a lot. Some researchers claim to do it in a few minutes, or over the telephone, or online. How do they get away with that?

Well, for three reasons, I think. First, differences readily match common social observations, much as a model of the universe once matched everyone's experience of sun and stars going around the earth. In the case of intelligence, we sense it comes in grades, with people arranged on a kind of ladder. Second – and partly because of that – it's been easy for scientists to propose a *natural* ladder; that is, intelligence based on our biological make-up. That makes differences real and immutable. Third, IQ testing became influential because it's been so useful as a socially practical tool. Psychologists have boasted about that for a long time.

Indeed, there's a long history behind all of that. Proving that the intelligence we 'see' socially is perceived accurately, and is biologically inevitable, was the task of polymath Herbert Spencer. Writing in utilitarian Victorian Britain of the 1850s, one biographer described him as 'the single most famous European intellectual' of his time. Spencer did try to create a theory of intelligence, but didn't get far. He was sure, however, that individual and group differences must originate in the physiology of the brain, and due more 'to the completion of the cerebral organization, than to the individual experiences'. 'From this law', he went on, 'must be deducible all the phenomena of unfolding intelligence, from its lowest to its highest grades'.

Spencer's method was still theoretical. He read Darwin, and coined the term 'survival of the fittest'. That idea was later to inspire a wider eugenics movement favouring policies like selective breeding. From common observation he told us that 'the minds of the inferior human races, cannot respond to relations of even moderate complexity'. By the same token, helping the poor and weak in British society flew in the face of nature, he said – they should be allowed to perish. That's also practical, in a way, if rather blunt. But sharper tools were on the horizon.

An Unnatural Measure

Gentleman scientist Sir Francis Galton followed much of Spencer's drift. He was, in addition, very practically minded. In possession of a fortune (inherited), Galton was able to indulge many interests. Travels in Africa in the 1850s had already convinced him of the mental inferiority of its natives. He had read Charles Darwin's theory, conversed with Spencer, and became convinced that there is something he called 'natural ability'. It varies substantially among people, he argued, just like height and weight, and is distributed like the bell-shaped curve. Later he observed that members of the British establishment were often related to each other. That convinced him that differences in intelligence must lie in biological inheritance, which also implied that society could be improved through eugenics, or selective breeding programmes. However, he realised, that would need some measure 'for the indications of superior strains or races, and in so favouring them that their progeny shall outnumber and gradually replace that of the old one'.

Galton was amazingly energetic and inventive. He believed that differences in natural ability, being innate, must lie in neurological efficiency, or the 'physiology of the mind' – functions obviously hidden and unidentified. He reasoned, however, that responses to simple sensorimotor tests could provide a window on those hidden differences. He even set up a special laboratory and got people to pay for the fun: reaction times, speed of hand motions, strength of grip, judgements of length, weight, and many others, which all provided the data he sought.

Of course, individuals varied in their scores. But how could he convince people that they were really differences in the unseen intelligence? He already had an idea: 'the sets of measures should be compared with an independent estimate of the man's powers', he said. The individuals' social status and reputation were what he had in mind. As he put it in *Hereditary Genius* (1883), 'my argument is to show that high reputation is a pretty accurate test of high ability'.

And that was it: a numerical surrogate of human worth, of 'strains and races', in a few quick tests of sensation, speed, and motion. If you're thinking about it, though, you might see some suspicious circularity in the logic and want to ask Sir Francis a few questions, like:

- How do you know that reputation is a good indication of natural ability (and not, for example, a consequence of social background)?

Possible answer: It's the only one I can employ (he actually said that) – or, more honestly, we don't really know.

- If you know in advance who is more or less intelligent, why do you need the test?

Possible answer: For mass testing. Also, because numbers look objective and scientific.

- If the tests are chosen to agree with what you already know, how can it possibly be more accurate?

Possible answer: It logically cannot be; but it looks as if it is.

These questions refer to the 'validity' of a test. Does it measure what it claims to measure? Or do we really know what score differences are differences in? Those questions have hung over intelligence testing like a dark cloud ever since. In this chapter, I hope to show you how IQ testers have dealt with it, and how that has entailed a very special understanding of intelligence. To get a better idea of validity, though, let's briefly compare the strategy with real tests of physiology, as in biomedical tests.

Physiological Testing

Like psychologists, real physiologists need to describe hidden causes of observed differences, especially in disease conditions. So they have long pored over whatever fluids, excretions, secretions, or expectorants they could coax from the insides to compare with outer symptoms.

Urinalysis was practised even in Ancient Greece, in the time of Hippocrates. In the Middle Ages, flasks and charts were carried by all respectable physicians, duly called 'pisse prophets', to assist diagnosis. Colour charts, used well into the nineteenth century, as well as notes on smell (and sometimes taste!) were the first attempts at standardised tests of physiology. Diabetic urine was noted for its 'exceeding sweetness'. It's thought that this is where the expression 'taking the piss' stems from.

Of course, the tests were rough and ready. But validity improved for a simple reason. Scientific research painstakingly revealed the true nature of the internal functions, including the many detailed steps in urine production, where they can go wrong, and how that is reflected in the chosen markers. So today we have a formidable array of valid tests of physiological functions. We can reliably rate differences in the measure on the 'outside' – even the colour of urine – to the unseen functional differences on the 'inside'. We can understand what variations in cholesterol measures mean. Likewise with blood pressure readings; why a white blood cell count is an index of levels of internal infection; and why a roadside breathalyser reading corresponds fairly accurately with level of alcohol consumption.

'We Classify'

It turned out that Galton's test didn't work, anyway. Differences between upper class and tradesmen, having experienced contrasting conditions in development, would have been unsurprising. But they turned out to be tiny. For example, reaction time to sound was 0.147 versus 0.152 seconds. For 'highest audible sound', Galton recorded 17,530 versus 17,257 vibrations per second. But what about intellectual differences? In the USA, doctoral student Clark Wissler tried to correlate results from Galton's tests with academic grades of university students. There was virtually no correlation between them. And the test scores did not even appear to correlate with each other. It is not possible, Wissler said, they could be valid measures of intelligence. The physiologists of the mind needed another approach.

It so happened that, around that time, the early 1900s, a psychologist in Paris was also devising psychological tests, though of a different kind and for a different purpose. Parisian schools were now admitting more children from poorer backgrounds, and some might struggle with unfamiliar demands. Alfred Binet was charged by the local school board to help identify those who might need help.

Like Galton, Binet devised series of quick questions and mental tasks. But he was looking for ones related to school learning rather than physiology. He got them, quite sensibly, from close observation of classroom activities, by devising short questions and tasks to reflect those activities, and then trying them out. Each item was deemed suitable, or not, according to two criteria: (1) whether the number of correct answers increased with age; and (2) whether a given child's performances matched teachers' judgements of his or her progress.

Binet and his colleague Henri Simon produced their first *Metrical Scale of Intelligence* in 1905. It contained 30 items, designed for children aged 3–12 years, arranged in order of difficulty. By 1911 the collection had expanded to 54 items. Here are some examples expected to be passable by two age groups:

Five-year olds:
- compare two weights;
- copy a square;

- repeat a sentence of 10 syllables;
- count four pennies;
- join the halves of a divided rectangle.

Ten-year olds:
- arrange five blocks in order of weight;
- copy drawings from memory;
- criticise an absurd statement;
- answer sentence-comprehension questions;
- use three given words into a sentence.

Average scores for each age group were calculated. The 'mental age' of individuals could then be worked out from how many items they could do. If a child achieved a score expected of six-year-olds, they would be said to have a mental age of six. A child passing them all would have a mental age of 12. Binet suggested that a deficit of two years or more between mental age and chronological age indicated that help was needed. Finally, in 1912, the German psychologist William Stern proposed the use of the ratio of mental age to chronological age to yield the now familiar intelligence quotient, or IQ:

$$IQ = \frac{\text{mental age}}{\text{chronological age}} \times 100.$$

So IQ was born. But it is important to stress the narrow, practical, purpose of Binet's test: 'Psychologists do not measure . . . we classify', he said. However, it had an unintended, but hugely portentous, quality. By its nature it produced different scores for different social classes and 'races'. Galton's followers soon claimed Binet's to be the test of innate intelligence they had been looking for. Translations appeared in many parts of the world, especially in the USA. Binet himself condemned the perversion of his tests as 'brutal pessimism'.

Original Mental Endowment

In the USA, Henry H. Goddard translated the Binet–Simon test into English in 1908, and found it useful for assessing the 'feebleminded'. As a eugenicist, Goddard worried about the degeneration of the 'race' (and nation) by the mentally handicapped, and also by the waves of new immigrants from

Southern and Eastern Europe. He was commissioned to administer the test to arrivals at the immigration reception centre on Ellis Island. Test scores famously suggested that 87 per cent of the Russians, 83 per cent of the Jews, 80 per cent of the Hungarians, and 79 per cent of the Italians were feebleminded. Demands for immigration laws soon followed.

Lewis Terman, a professor at Stanford University, developed another translation of Binet's test in 1916. He enthused over the way it could help clear 'high-grade defectives' off the streets, curtail 'the production of feeblemindedness', and eliminate crime, pauperism, and industrial inefficiency. By using his IQ test, he said, we could 'preserve our state for a class of people worthy to possess it'. Binet's screen for a specific category thus became scores of the genetic worth of people in general. 'People do not fall into two well defined groups, the "feeble minded" and the "normal"', Terman said. 'Among those classed as normal vast individual differences exist in original mental endowment.' He, too, called for eugenic reproduction controls, which soon followed. Galton's programme had found its measure.

Mass Testing

Terman's test was applied to individuals, one at a time. During World War I, however, the US Army wanted to test recruits in large numbers from many different backgrounds. A group led by Robert Yerkes constructed two pencil-and-paper tests: one for those who could read and write English; the other for those who could not. These were quite ingenious, including tasks like tracing through a maze, completing a picture with a part missing, and comparing geometrical shapes. Up to 60 recruits could be tested at a time, taking 40–50 minutes. In *Army Mental Tests*, published in 1920, Clarence Yokum and Robert Yerkes claimed that the test was 'definitely known … to measure native intellectual ability'.

These group tests set the scene for mass IQ testing in populations generally, and for the spread of the ideology underlying it. Up to the early 1930s the IQ message became useful in the USA in the passing of compulsory sterilisation laws, immigration laws, and the banning of 'inter-racial' marriage. Hitler's ministers in Nazi Germany were impressed by America's IQ testing regimes, and its eugenics policies. They took the message away with even more deadly consequences, as we all know.

And in Britain

In Britain, the new intelligence tests were just as energetically promoted. Eugenics movements were popular, and, in 1911, a report to the *Board of Education* recommended their use for the identification of 'mental defectives'. By the late 1930s psychologists like Cyril Burt were urging their use in the British 11+ exam. 'It is possible at a very early age', they advised, 'to predict with accuracy the ultimate level of a child's intellectual power', and that 'different children . . . require (different) types of education'.

Since then, IQ testing has developed rapidly into the huge enterprise it is today. But constant controversy has hinged on the same burning question. Do IQ tests really measure what they claim to measure – even if we aren't sure what that is? It's important to see how IQ testers have dealt with the question, and how they have dodged it.

Validity Vacuum

In his book *IQ and Human Intelligence*, Nicholas Macintosh stated: 'If you are trying to devise a test that will measure a particular trait . . . it will surely help to have a psychological theory specifying the defining features of the trait, to ensure that the test maps on to them.' That means being clear about what differences on the 'outside' (the measure) really mean in terms of differences on the 'inside'. That's what we expect of modern physiological and biomedical tests, after all. Such mapping is called 'construct validity'. As mentioned earlier, simple definitions do not do that.

Lewis Terman used previously translated items from Binet's test, but added many more of similar types: memory span, vocabulary, word definition, general knowledge, and so on. Now called the Stanford–Binet, the test soon became the standard on both sides of the Atlantic. Like Binet's test items, they obviously tended to reflect school learning and a literary/numerical mindset, itself related to social background. But there is no systematic attempt at construct validity.

As regards the *Army Mental Tests*, mentioned above, Yokum and Yerkes duly emphasised (on page 2!) that the test 'should have a high degree of validity as a test of intelligence'. But little more was said about it. Instead, correlations of scores with those on Terman's test, and with teachers' ratings, as well as social class, are given.

David Wechsler devised the *Adult Intelligence Scale* in 1939, and then the *Wechsler Scale for Children* in 1949. Wechsler had worked on the Army tests and used similar items. Through a number of revisions, these tests have rivalled the Stanford–Binet in popularity. As for validity, as psychologist Nicholas Mackintosh noted, 'Wechsler had little evidence [of] the validity of his tests', except their correlation with Stanford–Binet scores and teachers' ratings. He quotes Wechsler to say, 'How do we know that our tests are "good" measure of intelligence? The honest answer we can reply is that our own experience has shown them to be so.' As apology, Wechsler mentions only that the same applies 'to every other intelligence test'.

These are the most popular, and almost the 'gold standard', tests. A huge number of other IQ-type tests have been constructed, and I will refer to some below. But they are almost all collections of items closely related to school learning and literacy and numeracy. Testers almost always imply that they're measuring learning *ability*, not simply learning. What that is has not been made clear. If you get the chance, have a look at the test manuals and search for any claims about test validity. What you will almost always get is reference to one or other of four substitutes for it. Let us look at these in turn.

Score Patterns

IQ test items are devised by individual psychologists introspectively, according to the cognitive processes they imagine will be invoked. They are then included or rejected in a test after exhaustive trial-and-error procedures known as item analysis. The aim is to end up with a pattern of average scores that match expectations of individual differences in intelligence. An item is included if, as seen in trials, it more or less contributes to such a pattern. Otherwise it is rejected. Although the pattern is thus 'built in', it is then taken to confirm test validity.

For example, test constructors have assumed that intelligence, as a 'biological' trait, should be distributed like physical traits, according to the bell-shaped curve (Figure 1.1). The pattern was achieved by Lewis Terman, after preliminary trials, by a simple device: rejecting items that proved to be either too easy or too difficult for most people. The practise has continued, and the results have been taken to confirm test validity, instead of being an artefact of test construction. In fact, many physiological variables, including many in the brain, are not distributed like that (see Chapter 6).

Test items are also selected such that progressively more of each age group respond correctly. That makes scores resemble those of a simple physical trait such as height or foot size. However, the school-related content of many items ensures that average test scores indeed increase with age – as desired – and then steadily decline thereafter (Figure 1.2). Even today, researchers worry about the declining average intelligence of adults, and are looking

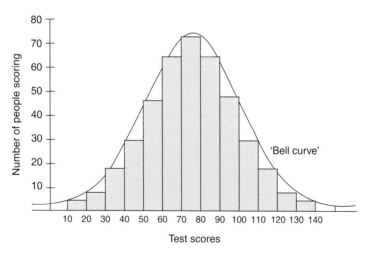

Figure 1.1   The famous bell-shaped curve 'built in' to the IQ test. Raw scores usually get converted statistically to IQs with a mean of 100.

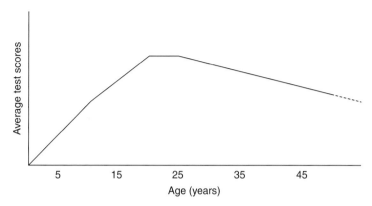

Figure 1.2   Rise and fall of IQ test scores with age.

(unsuccessfully) for the neural bases of it. But it's only a side-effect of the method of test construction.

The problem could, of course, be solved, by introducing items that older people are better at. In such ways, sex differences evident in the original Stanford–Binet test were equalised by introducing, in later revisions, new items on which boys did better than girls, or vice versa. Other psychologists have shown how social class and 'racial' differences could be eliminated (or even reversed) in exactly the same way. In all these ways we find 'test validity' inferred from score patterns that are actually consequences of test construction.

Scores Agree – It Must Be '*g*'

We all appreciate how entities that change (i.e. variables) can sometimes change together, or co-vary: for example, season and daytime temperature, or shoe size and hand size. In the late nineteenth century, Karl Pearson devised a statistical measure of such co-variation. His 'correlation coefficient', widely used ever since, ranges from 0 to 1 (0.0–1.0) according to the degree of co-variation. Psychologists often warn about inferring causes from correlations: the price of coffee correlates with global warming but does not cause it. But they also have a habit of ignoring it. That has been an issue running throughout the history of IQ.

People who do well on one kind of mental test (such as an intelligence test or school test) tend to do well on others, and vice versa. British psychologist Charles Spearman had noted that in the early 1900s. He suggested that the correlations must be caused by the single underlying factor proposed by Galton: a 'General Intelligence' that he also called 'g'. The correlations were not perfect (around 0.6 for school subjects). So Spearman suggested that individual differences were also partly due to differences in 'special' factors, meaning ability at some particular cognitive tasks (such as maths or writing).

Such correlations are taken by leading IQ testers as proof of test validity – that the tests are really invoking a real and common intelligence factor. But that is a causal inference from the correlations, not a fact. It might be due to something else, and there have been big disagreements about that. As just described, test items are selected according to the designer's preconceptions and ingenuity. So, some tests are constructed to emphasise the unitary factor g as causing most individual differences; others emphasise the special or 'group' factors, such as 'verbal' or 'visuo-spatial' abilities. That has caused much debate about the 'structure' of intelligence, as if the different score patterns are saying something about internal processes rather than test construction.

Behind it all is a tacit model of the mind as a kind of machine. Even today, Spearman's g is said to reflect individual differences in some kind of 'energy', 'power', 'capacity', or even 'speed of processing'. The special or group factors are treated as if they are components in the machine. People vary, that is, according to the 'strengths' of their components. Again, we don't know what they are or how they work. The names they are given – such as memory, verbal, mathematical – simply describe the 'look' of respective items, not real cognitive functions. Yet correlation patterns in a test are frequently presented as evidence of test validity. We should not be fooled by them.

I will be reminding readers frequently of this 'mechanical' model of the human mind. It underlies much of what is wrong in research and ideas about intelligence.

Predictive Validity

By far the most quoted source of test validity consists of associations with other aspects of achievement. '[T]he measurement of intelligence ... is a reasonably good predictor of grades at school, performance at work, and many other aspects of success in life.' So said a report for the American Psychological Association in 2012. It is a well-rehearsed mantra, and IQ testers readily join the chorus line.

Does that really tell us what is being measured? Things are not so simple. There *are* correlations between individuals' IQs and their school performances. But IQ test items tend to be selected *because* they are related to school knowledge and learning. They are, to a large extent, measuring the same learning. A correlation between the two is self-fulfilling, and hardly an independent index of test validity.

Another problem with the argument is that the associations diminish over time, outside the narrow confines of early school learning. In the UK, IQ predicts GCSE (General Certificate of Secondary Education) performances in tests taken at around 16 years old. But the latter only moderately predict A-level performances two years later, which, in turn, only very moderately predict university performance (see Chapter 9). That doesn't suggest we're measuring a very robust 'intelligence'.

IQ scores are also statistically associated with occupational level, salary, and so on. But level of entry to the job market is largely determined by school attainment. That's another self-fulfilling pseudo-validity. But what about job *performance*? For nearly a century, in fact, hundreds of studies have tried to assess how much IQ predicts job performance. But only very weak correlations (around 0.2) could be found. IQ testers, however, tend to appeal to the remarkable 'corrections' hammered out of the originals by the complex statistical manoeuvres of industrial psychologists Frank Schmidt, John Hunter, and their associates in the 1980s. The corrections involved 'pooling' all the available results and have attracted many criticisms – for very good reasons.

The original studies tended to be old, some from the 1920s, and related to particular jobs, companies, and locations, mainly in the USA. Many were performed in rough-and-ready circumstances, with only small samples. And many of the tests were not even IQ tests: reading tests, memory tests, simple vocabulary or English tests, judgement of speed, and other 'aptitude' tests – in fact, dozens of anything looking remotely like a mental test. It seems a travesty to call these 'general ability tests' as Schmidt and others do. Moreover, the statistical corrections required crucial information about test reliabilities, measurement errors, score ranges, and so on. In many cases that information was not available, so had to be estimated using more assumptions. Yet these corrections have been extremely influential in backing up supposed test validity. Those who continue to rely on them really should look at the datasets more closely.

In fact, job performance is difficult to assess objectively, and has almost always been based on supervisor ratings. Those tend to be subjective, and based on inconsistent criteria. Age, height, ethnic group, and facial attractiveness have all been shown to sway judgements. And – as we surely all know – performance can vary drastically from time to time, in different contexts, work environments, and how long individuals have spent on the job. In sum, the idea that IQ tests are valid measures of intelligence because they predict educational and job performance is debatable. The bottom line, anyway, is that none of these so-called test validities are clear about what the measures are measuring. So let's have a closer look at that.

Differences in What?

It is not difficult to find examples of IQ test items in magazines and online. To the general public they can seem impressive and convincing. They can look as if they definitely need complex mental processing. The variety, hatched through the ingenuity of item designers, is itself impressive: word meanings, synonyms, block puzzles, identifying shapes; there's hundreds of them. So only a few examples can be considered here.

Many require general knowledge, such as: What is the boiling point of water? Who wrote Hamlet? In what continent is Egypt? These fall under the category of 'verbal intelligence'. But they surely demand little more than factual knowledge obviously learned, and, as such, related to background opportunities for doing so.

Most items require some use of words and numbers, such as recall of a short string of digits like 5, 2, 4, 9, 6, or of words like dog, camera, train, animal, job. They are read out to be recalled five minutes later as a measure of memory. Others are classified as 'verbal comprehension', such as:

Which single letter completes the following words? CA*; *US; RU*Y; *OTH.

'Verbal reasoning' items are deemed to be particularly important, and usually include verbal analogies such as:

Horse is to foal as Cow is to (calf; to be chosen from the given options).

These also come in nonverbal forms, as shown in Figure 1.3.

Indeed, whole tests have been based on such 'analogical reasoning items', and it's instructive to take a special look at them. In his book *Innate* (2018), Kevin Mitchell describes analogical reasoning as 'at the very heart of intelligence'. That argument, too, seems convincing until we consider the way that so much of everyday human communication and activity utilises analogical reasoning:

> 'His bark is worse than his bite.'
> 'Letting the tail wag the dog.'
> 'The harder you shake the pack the easier it will be for some cornflakes to get to the top.' (Boris Johnson on IQ and schooling.)

Biblical proverbs, sermons, and parables use them a lot (I seem to remember something about rich folk, heaven, a camel, and the eye of a needle). So does

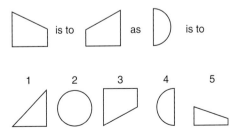

Figure 1.3 Typical nonverbal analogy item.

much of everyday humour. As I will explain in other parts of this book, analogy formation and recognition are aspects of the general pattern abstraction that takes place even in simple organisms. Indeed, Mitchell himself uses analogies to get across certain points:

> Sexual selection [e.g. females being choosy about partners] can act [on males] like an escalating arms race. (p. 157)

> The [resting] brain is like a car sitting with its engine running, just idling. (p. 28)

When authors use analogies in that way, they do so with an obvious assumption: that the analogy will be understandable *through familiarity*, from experience. So, it seems reasonable to ask why we would assume the opposite with IQ tests: that they reveal something *other* than familiarity? That's like swallowing camels and straining at gnats. (And there's another one.)

In fact, many studies have now shown, even in young children, how ability to do specific analogical reasoning items does depend on familiarity with the relations bound up in them, rather than a hypothetical mental 'strength' or 'power'. They seem to be so widely included in IQ tests for no other reason than that they reliably discriminate between social classes – which, of course, gives the whole game away. Such black box, mechanical thinking also exposes the point made by Linda Gottfredson in 1997, that 'We lack systematic task analyses of IQ tests.'

It's worth applying that caution to other nonverbal items, which are very popular. These include identifying missing parts of pictures (e.g. a face with its nose missing); tracing routes through mazes; counting boxes in a stack (with some of them hidden behind others); and so on. By far the favourites, however, are matrix items (Figure 1.4). *Raven's Matrices* tests are made up entirely of such items. Again, it is instructive to give them further consideration.

In order to solve a matrix, test-takers need to work out the rules dictating changes across rows and down columns. These are mostly changes to size, position, or number of elements. The difficulty seems to depend on the number of rules to be identified and the dissimilarity of elements to be

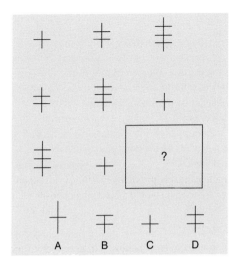

Figure 1.4 A simple matrix item. Test-takers have to complete the matrix by choosing from the alternatives underneath.

compared. A tremendous mystique has developed around them. Their appearance suggests that they really are getting at basic differences in cognitive ability, free from any cultural or other background influence.

In fact, a little further analysis shows that 'Raven IQ' is just as dependent on familiarity, itself varying with social background, as the analogies items. The manipulation of elements (e.g. words, numbers) in two-dimensional arrays on paper or computer screens is very common in many jobs and family backgrounds, and less so in others. It figures prominently in record sheets, tables with rows and columns giving totals and subtotals, spreadsheets, timetables, and so on, as well as ordinary reading material. These nearly all require the reading of symbols from top left to bottom right, and additions, subtractions, and substitutions across columns and down rows. Familiarity with such relations and procedures varies significantly across cultures and social classes. For example, Asian cultures that read from right to left have difficulty with them. That suggests what is really being tested.

Real-Life Complexity

We can't be sure what cognitive processes are really being compared in IQ tests. On the other hand, it can be claimed that typical IQ test items are remarkably *un*-complex in comparison to the complexity of cognitive processing nearly all of us use every day. Ordinary, everyday, social life is more complex than we think. As Linda Gottfredson also explained, 'other individuals are among the most complex, novel, changing, active, demanding, and unpredictable objects in our environments'. The mental activity needed to deal with real life tends to be a great deal more complex than that required by IQ test items, including those in the Raven.

Some studies have set up simulated factories, tailor's shops, or public services, where participants have to control several variables at once (staff numbers, input costs, and so on) to maximise production. Reported associations with IQ have tended to be weak. In 1986 psychologists Stephen Ceci and Jeffrey Liker reported their famous study of betting at a racecourse. They found gamblers' predictions of odds to be a sophisticated cognitive process. It involved taking account of up to 11 variables, with complex interactions between them. Individuals' accuracy at such predictions was unrelated to their IQ test scores.

Highly complex cognition is already evident in pre-school children. Developmental psychologist Erno Téglás and colleagues argue, as I will do many times later, that 'many organisms can predict future events from the statistics of past experience'. That means integrating many sources of information 'to form rational expectations about novel situations, never directly experienced'. We do this all the time in ordinary social situations (think about driving in a strange town). But what Téglás and colleagues found is that 'this reasoning is surprisingly rich, powerful, and coherent even in preverbal infants'.

Much other evidence shows how different people, in different circumstances, develop different ways of thinking and feeling. These are even reflected in brain networks, as we shall see in Chapter 6. Being cognitively intelligent means different things for different people in many different places. As the European Human Behaviour and Evolution Association warned in a statement in 2020, 'Even those IQ tests which claim to be culture-neutral . . . rely on modes of thinking which are routinely embedded in Western education systems (e.g. analysing 2-dimensional stimuli), but not reflective of skills and learning experiences of a large proportion of the global population.'

It is perfectly reasonable to ask, then, are IQ tests testing for mental 'strength' or familiarity? The latter will vary for many reasons other than innate endowments. Indeed, I will be presenting much evidence that those we label as intelligent – or bright or smart or whatever – tend to be those culturally 'like us'. In speaking the same language, they are using the same cognitive rules of engagement, and similar conceptual models of the world. Engagement with ease and confidence also creates the illusion of underlying mental strength or power.

Familiarity and Class

Familiarity with items, as in analogies and matrices, will mostly vary with social background. As a 2017 review by psychologist Natalie Brito found, the specific language and numerical skills needed for IQ tests are closely related to social class background. So it's not so much individual strength, power, or capacity that is being described in IQ differences as the demographics of the society in which they have lived.

That explains why *average* IQ scores have increased enormously across generations in all societies where records are available: about 15 points per generation. It has been called the 'Flynn effect', after James Flynn, one of the researchers first reporting it. IQ theorists are still puzzled about it. It could not be due to hypothetical genetic changes over such a short time. Nor is it likely to be due to general improvements in simple speed, capacity, or strength. The effect does correspond, however, with massive expansion of middle-class occupational roles, and reduction of working class roles. More and more people have simply become more familiar with the acquired numerical and literary skills of the middle class.

Not Intelligence

IQ test performances will also vary for reasons that have little to do with cognition or learning ability. Some children will be motivated or 'pushed' by parents to acquire the knowledge, and the skills of numeracy and literacy, that figure in IQ tests. So it is not surprising that IQ also varies with degrees of parental support and encouragement. That will also tend to affect performance on *all* tests – which may be the real basis of the mysterious 'general intelligence', or '*g*', mentioned above. Also, as anyone might expect, levels of self-confidence, stress, motivation, and anxiety, and general physical and mental vigour, all affect education, job, and cognitive test performances. Such factors are not spread randomly across a population. They will be closely associated with social class, and I will explore them further in Chapter 8.

Finally, although we are led to believe that IQ is a fixed attribute of an individual, that's far from the case. Of course, if individuals' social status and test-relevant experiences don't change, neither will their proficiency on IQ tests, even over many years or even decades. That simply reflects continuity of social class membership. On the other hand, IQ test performance is demonstrably boosted by practice. Testing of the same individual at different times can show variations of as much as 30 points (over an average score of 100). IQs can improve with schooling, as just mentioned. Also, children adopted into middle-class homes from an early age have IQs, on average, 15 points higher than those not adopted. Other test-related experiences, such as computer games or even music training, can also boost IQ scores.

Other Ideas

The IQ view of intelligence continues to dominate biology and psychology. But some psychologists, conscious of its problems, have tried to present alternatives. An entertaining account of some of these is given in science journalist David Robson's *The Intelligence Trap*, mostly based on the shortcomings of IQ testing (though without further analysis).

In *Multiple Intelligences* (1984) and *Extraordinary Minds* (1997), Howard Gardner has debunked the concept of *g*. Instead, he suggests there are 'specialised intelligences' such as linguistic intelligence, logico-mathematical intelligence, spatial intelligence, musical intelligence, and so on. In his more recent work, Gardner has extended his original list of 7 to 11, and suggests the list will grow. He doesn't give details of cognitive processes, but speculates that each 'intelligence' has its own peculiar computational mechanisms, based on a distinct neural architecture. Intelligences, he says, also differ in strength from person to person. That explains, he suggests, why all children excel in one or two domains, while remaining mediocre or downright backward in others.

All that aligns with those who intuitively sense individual 'talents' in children. The problem is, where do they come from? Gardner also passes the question over to biology. He says that they are predetermined through genetic programmes. The specified structures will develop even in widely varying circumstances or environmental experiences, but individuals will vary in their 'intelligences' through inherited differences in those programmes. Thus, while appealing for its broader view, Gardner's theoretical foundations remain tentative and undeveloped. Some see his 'theory' as just a 'naming' exercise – identifying areas of expertise in individuals without describing what any one actually is, or how it works or develops.

Psychologist Robert Sternberg has, for many years, expressed dismay at the narrowness of the concept of *g*. On his website in 2020 he says that 'we no longer can afford to define intelligence merely as *g* or IQ. Doing so has been a disaster – literally, not merely figuratively.' He has been developing a 'triarchic' theory of intelligence, based on three wider attributes:

1. analytical thinking is that ability assumed in traditional IQ tests;
2. creative ability, which forms the basis of imagination and innovation; and
3. practical intelligence, which is the ability to plan and execute decisions.

Sternberg says people vary in these different domains, and they influence decision-making and success in life. He has also attempted to develop tests for them. For example, in regard to 'practical intelligence', individuals are presented with problems relevant to their work context. He argues that those tests offer better predictions of university grades and occupational success than basic IQ tests. The theory has been lauded in some quarters for identifying intelligent individuals otherwise missed. But that does not really tell us what individuals have got and how they got it. However, we must look forward to Sternberg's forthcoming *Adaptive Intelligence* (due 2021). Forward notices say it involves 'dramatic reappraisal and reframing of ...

a fatally-flawed, outdated conception of intelligence'. It may be that what I have to say in Chapters 8 and 9, in particular, will be in some agreement with that.

There have been many other alternative views. In my view, they are adjuncts to the mechanical IQ view of intelligence differences. Some are refreshing, but do not get to the root of the matter of what intelligence is, how it evolved, and how it develops in individuals. What intelligence 'is' remains implicit (or, as Sternberg says, 'tacit') rather than explicit. That requires the more radical approach attempted in most of this book.

Use of IQ Tests

No one can criticise the medieval 'pisse prophets' for trying to help the physically distressed. The same applies to attempts to identify individuals in need of psychological help today. That was the intention of Binet through his original test: a purely pragmatic tool, without prejudgment of future intelligence, or even a theory of it. Today, many clinicians and other psychologists claim to find some IQ-type test items useful in helping children and adults in just that way. For example, some 'visuo-spatial' tests may help diagnose early Alzheimer's disease. Some 'verbal' tests might identify specific problems with reading, and so on. And you may have read that the Wechsler Digit Symbol test is a 'neuropsychological test' sensitive to brain damage, dementia, and so on. But we must also be aware of their limitations.

We can describe an item by appearance, but we don't really know what is happening 'in' the brain or cognitive system. That may lead users astray sometimes, as happened with medieval physicians. For example, as with all cognitive testing, performance is subject to the multitude of contextual and social background factors mentioned above. Test-takers who are illiterate, have little education, or lack cognitive confidence will show significantly lower performance on *all* cognitive assessment tests without lacking in learning ability at all.

Nevertheless, such specific uses may also be helpful in very complex circumstances, and they may well be useful in the long-term research needed to construct better theories of intelligence (which is what much of the rest of this book is about). What we cannot do is what happened as soon as the Binet–Simon tests were translated and used in Anglo-American contexts: that is, claim to have a measure of general intelligence – and genetic worth – in whole populations. Alas, that is a mistake being widely repeated today.

Back to Physiology

Galton's followers have always tried to identify differences in intelligence with physiology. As educational psychologist Arthur Jensen put it in the 1980s, 'the g factor is so thoroughly enmeshed in brain physiology' as to really be 'a property of the brain as a whole'. Much of the rest of this book will show that real biological systems are nothing like the 'physiology' those psychologists imagine. Here's a glimpse of why.

Today, there are thousands of physiological tests, all external 'biomarkers' of clearly modelled internal differences. One of the most striking things about them, though, is the extremely wide ranges of variation within which normal, adequate function seems to operate. The following list presents what are 'normal' measures of physiological functions in a standard full blood count. Only deviations outside these wide limits suggest abnormality:

- red blood cells: 4.5–6.5 trillion cells per litre;
- white cells (for immunity): 4.0–11.0 billion cells per litre;
- platelets (for clotting): 140–400 billion per litre;
- lymphocytes (guiding immune response): 1.5–4.0 billion per litre;
- vitamin B12 (for a wide range of processes): 150–1,000 nanograms per litre;
- serum ferritin (levels of stored iron): 12.0–250 micrograms per litre;
- serum folate (involved in DNA and red blood cell production): 2.0–18.8 micrograms per litre;
- serum urea (indicates kidney function): 2.5–7.8 micromoles per litre;
- alkaline phosphatase (indicates liver function): 30–130 units per litre.

These are very wide, yet normal, variations. Within them the system functions well enough. In a different context, the biophysicist Nicolas Rashevsky introduced the term 'the principle of adequate design'. I think it fits very well in this context, too. Real physiology is nothing like the simplistic bell-curve model. It is a dynamic, interactive system of processes that tend to mutually compensate for each other. Indeed, I will show in Chapter 4 that physiology is, itself, an intelligent system. Huge variation observed is little guide to what lies beneath – which is what most of this book is about.

2 In the Genes?

Whether they believe in IQ or not, most people sense that individual differences in intelligence are substantial and at least partly 'genetic'. The nature–nurture debate about the origins of such differences goes back a long way; at least as far as the philosopher-scientists of Ancient Greece. And most people have probably adopted common-sense views about it for just as long. It is evident today in popular cliches: our genetic blueprints set levels of potential, while nurture determines how much of it is reached; individual differences result from *both* genes and environments; genes and environments interact to determine individual differences; and so on.

Most of this chapter is about how biologists and psychologists have studied the origins of such differences. I hope to show that reaching out to biology has been far more concerned with vindicating a particular view of individual differences than what intelligence really is. In consequence, intelligence has been researched biologically rather as the agriculturalist studies crop growing, or the animal breeder seeks to boost specific traits. Individual differences have been treated as variation in a physical 'strength' or 'power', like the speed of greyhounds or the spring of thoroughbred hurdlers. It has left us with narrow views of both genes and environments, and little understanding or agreement about what intelligence really is.

At the present time, there is something almost evangelical about the new faith in genes. For several decades many IQ testers have called themselves 'behaviour geneticists'. Now they're swinging DNA at us like a demolition ball, and creating a frenzy in the popular media: 'Being rich and successful is in your

DNA' (*Guardian*, 12 July 2018); 'A new genetic test could help determine children's success' (*Newsweek*, 10 July 2018); 'Our fortune telling genes' predict our future intelligence (several places); and so on.

There is little modesty about it. Authors marshal every hyperbole: breakthrough, game-changer, exciting advances, and so on. Promises of a 'new genetics' of intelligence are thrown like confetti. Critics are condemned as 'gene deniers', 'science-deniers', or even (in a further hint of ideology) 'race-deniers', while the message has caught fund-raisers' eyes, pervaded institutions, and reached government advisers and prime ministers.

Why the exuberance? 'Mountains of data', say the IQ champions, from lots of new studies. What that means, in fact, is mountains of *correlations*, from questionable measures using statistical models based on unlikely assumptions.

In this chapter I look at the real nature of those data and the statistical models through which they are filtered and formed. They are debatable, but they are also instructive about the understanding of intelligence underlying them. In Chapter 3 I will lay the foundations of a real theory of real intelligence. Its many ramifications fill the rest of the book.

An Agricultural Model

That 'something' is transmitted from parents to offspring, that can make differences in us – in particular traits – is obvious. There is also some predictability about it. Farmers and animal and crop breeders have exploited this fact for millennia, and we have much to thank them for. The apparent transmission is not straightforward, like the social inheritance of wealth. Offspring bear both similarities and differences to parents, and each other. She may have her mother's nose, but maybe not her mother's eyes or mouth, rather her father's – or even features different from both parents. We settle for terms of approximation like 'family resemblance'. Sometimes the effects of environment on some traits, as with nutrition and exercise on growth, are equally obvious.

The question for farmers and breeders – and what has also dominated the subject of human intelligence – was how to distinguish effects of different genes from those of different environments. In agricultural circles, in the early twentieth century, the issue had become a pressing economic one, and became called 'heritability'. Suppose variation in milk yield between cows is largely associated with genetic variation (there is a high 'heritability'). Then, it was argued, selecting for breeding those individuals who already exhibit high milk yield may boost the average yield in offspring. If the variation is estimated to be mainly due to environmental variation (there is low heritability), selective breeding will not make much difference.

The solution to the issue was proposed by statistician Sir Ronald Fisher in a paper in 1918. We cannot actually 'see' the genes, but he argued that their effects may be inferred from the patterns of resemblances among known relatives. That seems logical enough, but such patterns can also come from environmental similarities and differences. How do we distinguish between them? Fisher's proposal was exceedingly bold because of the assumptions entailed.

Experiments by Gregor Mendel (discovered around 1900) later led to the realisation that genes come in pairs, one from each parent. These (the members of each pair) are called 'alleles' and, as received from parents, may be the same or different. Fisher's solution was basically as follows. Let's pretend that the alleles are equal in effect on variation, positive or negative. Also assume that individual differences are due to small effects of many genes and their respective alleles. Then, he suggested, the total 'genetic' effect is simply all those independent effects added together. That means assuming that genes vary like little electrical charges, positive or negative. Individual differences in a trait then reflect different sums of those charges (Figure 2.1).

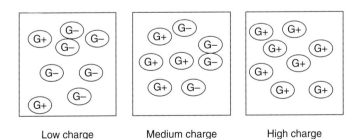

Low charge   Medium charge   High charge

Figure 2.1   Genetic effects for three individuals in Fisher's model. More positive (+) charges means a higher trait score, and vice versa for negative (−) charges.

That makes a very simple picture. The 'strength' of an individual's intelligence, say, lies in the particular permutation of strong or weak alleles (at least of those alleles that make a difference). So behaviour geneticists speak of 'intelligence-enhancing alleles' and 'intelligence-depleting alleles'. More importantly, the picture can be used to determine heritability: how much different permutations are associated with differences in the trait. We now know that members of any species (humans or other animals) share the vast majority of their genes and their alleles. And most of those that vary don't make a difference to the trait anyway. What matters is those few that do and *how much* difference they make. That's heritability, usually expressed as a ratio between 0.0 and 1.0, or 0–100 per cent.

Of course, at that time, Fisher could not 'see' the genes, nor the degree to which individuals share them. But it could be estimated by comparing known relatives. In crops and animals, the degree of genetic sharing (or correlation) is known from their pedigrees, or breeding histories. In humans it is known from family relations. It was already known that identical twins (monozygotic, or MZ) come from one egg. So each pair can be presumed to share all their genes. If trait variation in a population is only due to different genes, MZ pairs aren't expected to differ in any of them. That is, correlations in trait measures should be around 1.0. Non-identical twins (dizygotic, or DZ) develop from two eggs. In consequence, they will vary, on average, in only half of those genes, so the trait correlation should be around 0.5. The same applies to parent–offspring pairs, and to pairs of non-twin siblings.

In summary, Fisher argued that the total genetic effect on variation – the heritability – can be estimated from genetic correlations among relatives. To be clear, if the estimated heritability for any trait is 1.0 (or 100 per cent), all the trait variation is associated with genetic variation. Anything less than 1.0 is attributed to environmental effects. Fisher himself was quite sure that 'figures for human measurements shows that there is little or no indication of non-genetic causes'.

In that way an agricultural model of individual differences descended on the understanding of humanity, including (as we shall see) our understanding of intelligence. It all sounds highly plausible, if not brilliant. But, even then,

Fisher noted possible complications. One of those was the assumption that genes exist rather as autonomous agents, dictating their difference-making effects. Another is the possibility that the gene effects might not just add together in that neat way. Effects of one gene might have effects on others (called *gene–gene interaction*). Also, their effects may be different in different environments (called *gene–environment interactions*).

The other complication is that trait differences are also affected by different environments. That's not a problem with cows in uniform fields, wheat in field plots, and so on. In those cases, effects of any environmental differences are assumed to be spread randomly across individuals; they don't sway the estimates one way or the other. But it's not so easy for humans in socially structured environments.

Fisher's heritability estimations did turn out to be useful in agricultural settings. More crucially, they laid the foundations of 'quantitative' genetics that swept biology and psychology. This still dominates today's thinking about sources of individual differences and how to estimate them, including recent DNA sequencing efforts. In the human context it has been epoch-making in drawing conclusions about nature and nurture, even guiding social and educational policy, as mentioned in Chapter 1.

Before taking you further down that highway, and seeing the busy traffic on it, I want to warn you of some more bumps. Readers should be aware that Fisher's model is still what passes for the 'genetics' of intelligence today. More recent research, however, has shown the foundations of the model – Fisher's assumptions – to be quite unsound, especially with more complex traits and functions. To give you some flavour of those doubts, here are some recent assessments by today's geneticists.

> [A]lthough quantitative genetics has proved highly successful in plant and animal breeding, it should be remembered that this success has been based on large pedigrees, well-controlled environments, and short-term prediction. When these methods have been applied to natural populations, even the most basic predictions fail, in large part due to poorly understood environmental factors ... Once we leave an experimental setting, we are effectively skating on thin ice. (Nick Barton and colleagues, 2019).

Quantitative genetics traces its roots back through more than a century of theory, largely formed in the absence of directly observable genotype data, and has remained essentially unchanged for decades ... the available molecular evidence indicates that biological systems are anything but additive and that we need to evaluate alternative ways of utilizing the new data to understand the function of the genome. (Ronald Nelson and colleagues, 2013)

Petter Portin and Adam Wilkins, in 2017, said that recent developments in genetics 'raise questions about both the utility of the concept of a basic "unit of inheritance" and the long implicit belief that genes are autonomous agents'. They noted that 'the classic molecular definition [is] obsolete', and that we need 'a new one based on contemporary knowledge'.

Significantly, too, reflecting on it all in 1951, Fisher himself questioned 'the so-called co-efficient [i.e. measure] of heritability, which I regard as one of those unfortunate short-cuts, which have often emerged in biometry for lack of a more thorough analysis of the data'.

Note that such realities – especially the now well-known interactions between gene products, and between them and different environments – compromise the very idea of heritability in complex traits. In particular, they indicate how 'heritability' is not a fixed aspect of individuals or of populations. But I will return to that later. Unfortunately, the idea has dominated the genetic study of human intelligence, and it still does. The IQ test was built around it. It pervades people's minds and popular culture about the nature–nurture effect on intelligence. And nearly all research in the genetics of IQ has consisted of a grim spinning out of its flawed preconceptions. What follows is a brief narrative on the methodological contortions needed to prop it up.

Cyril Burt's Twin Correlations

It was the determined educational psychologist Cyril Burt who brought Fisher's 'solution' into the domain of human mental abilities. Burt had already been active in IQ testing and was our 'adviser' on that game-changing education report mentioned in Chapter 1. He worked hard to apply Fisher's model to human intelligence, where control of environmental effects is not so easy. The simplest approach, he realised, would be to compare identical (MZ) twins who had been reared apart. By not sharing the same homes, neighbourhoods, and so on, that should eliminate – or so it seemed – any correlation between them due to environmental effects. The average correlation between such pairs of twins could, in theory, be a direct estimate of heritability.

In an influential set of papers in the 1950s, Burt claimed to have done just that and to have measured the IQs of twins reared apart. He arrived at an estimate of the heritability of IQ of 0.83. This means that, according to Burt, 83 per cent of individual differences in IQ is associated with genetic variation; only 17 per cent is associated with differences in their experiences.

Here, however, things get murky. Separated identical twins are relatively rare, and Burt seems to have been suspiciously lucky in finding so many. Starting with 15 in 1943, he added 6 pairs for a total of 21 in 1955, finishing with a total of 53 pairs in 1966. Strangely enough, the correlations he reported across all three sets remained exactly the same at 0.77. When psychologist Leon Kamin checked Burt's data and uncovered this anomaly in 1971, it was soon being described as 'The most sensational charge of scientific fraud this century.' Burt, by then, was dead and so unable to answer the charge. But his attempts to prove his strong hereditarian views are no longer recognised, even by supporters.

Other Twins Reared Apart

The Minnesota Study of Twins Reared Apart (MISTRA) was started in the late 1970s by psychologist Thomas Bouchard and colleagues. It ended with 81 pairs. The results, reported in prestigious journals and books, along with sensationalised magazine stories, shook scientific and general populations around the world. Bouchard and colleagues consistently reported high average correlations between pairs of twins in IQ and other tests, even though reared apart. That proves, they claimed, a heritability for IQ of 0.75. In 1993, psychologist Robert Plomin wrote about 'the powerful design of comparing twins reared apart', suggesting 'a heritability for g of 80%'. For psychologists, the results challenged some cherished views about human development. They inspired the controversial theory of Arthur Jensen and others on the causes of 'racial' and social class differences in intelligence.

However, there are many dubious aspects of these data, too. They have been subjected to forensic dissection by investigators like Leon Kamin and Jay Joseph. I focus on a few of the main problems, just to illustrate the scientific latitude common to this field.

Really Reared Apart?

The first and biggest problem concerns whether those twins were truly separated. The twins obviously shared an environment in the womb before birth. That can have lasting effects on development throughout life. But even after birth, this was no rigorous research design. Authors of the MISTRA study have said that arrangements for separation 'were sometimes informal', and that at least some of the pairs had spent as much as four years together before being separated. Many of the twins were simply brought up by grandparents, aunts, or cousins. And at least some of them had spent considerable amounts of time together. Further analyses reveal how the reports stretch the usual meaning of the word 'separated' beyond credulity.

There is also bias in other ways. In the age of opinion polls, we all know the importance of samples being representative. Twins generally tend to be self-selecting in any twin study. Many of the MISTRA twins were recruited through media appeals. Others were prompted to volunteer by friends or family, on the grounds that they were alike. And some knew each other prior to the study. As Jay Joseph has suggested, twins that volunteer may well be more similar than the average.

There have been other problems. They include inadequate or incomplete reporting of important details, and disallowing other investigators access to data (a fundamental tenet of research). I recommend Jay Joseph's famous blog for an exhaustive expose of these problems.

'Classical' Twin Studies

Separated twins are rare, so the main approach has been to compare pairs of MZ twins with pairs of DZ twins reared together. The degree to which their resemblances correspond with genetic resemblances (i.e. 1.0 versus 0.5) has also been used as an index of heritability. This is the 'classical twin method'. Since the 1930s, it has been the workhorse of those who want to estimate the heritability of IQ. There have been dozens of such studies and a consistent pattern of correlations has been reported for IQ: usually higher for MZ twins than for DZ twins. Some have combined correlational data into more complex statistical models, but make the same assumptions and end up saying much the same thing. The estimated heritability is reported to be around 0.5 – meaning 50 per cent of differences in IQ is associated with genetic differences.

Those are the results producing fanfares about genes and IQ, almost always inferring causal connections, and much hyperbole. 'The genetic contribution is not just statistically significant', says Plomin, 'it is massive. Genetics is the most important factor shaping who we are. It explains more of the psychological differences between us than everything else put together.' Other leading authors have followed in the wake. 'They show', says Kevin Mitchell in *Innate*, 'that genetic differences contribute substantially to individual differences in psychological traits'. In his book *Human Diversity*, Charles Murray says, 'no one who accepts the validity of twin studies finds reasons to dispute them'. Surely, the chorus enjoins, so many studies cannot be wrong?

More False Assumptions

But they are wrong, critics say: so wrong that the classical twin study can be described as one of the most misleading methods in the history of science. The main problem is this. Simply taking the difference between MZ and DZ correlations as an index of genetic effects makes a big assumption. This is that the environments experienced by MZ pairs are no more similar during development than for DZ pairs. The higher correlation between them could be due to that. It is called the equal environments assumption (EEA).

The assumption is demonstrably false, and the problem insurmountable. There is overwhelming evidence that parents, friends, and teachers *treat* MZ twins more similarly than DZ twins. MZ twins are more likely to dress alike, share bedrooms, friends, activities, and so on. In his major review of the EEA, Jay Joseph cites dozens of findings revealing very large differences between MZ and DZ pairs in experiences such as identity confusion, being brought up as a unit, being inseparable as children, and having an extremely strong level of closeness. It is also known that parents hold more similar expectations for their MZ than DZ twins. '[T]win researchers and their critics don't have to argue anymore about whether MZ and DZ environments are different, since almost everyone now agrees that they are different', Joseph says.

These effects will, of course, contribute to correlations between MZ twins. What is assumed to be 'genetic' may, in fact, be 'environmental' in origin. Some investigators claim to have assessed the importance of those treatment effects. But how can they? They would first need to know what the 'trait relevant' environments are. And they don't know that because they don't know what intelligence really is, nor how it develops. So the problem remains. Those who continue with twin studies just tend to ignore it.

But that's not the only problem. Usually overlooked is that parents often do the opposite with DZ twins. They tend to exaggerate any differences, leading to stereotypes taken up by family and friends, and 'lived up to' by the twins themselves. More crucially, many DZ twins consciously strive to make themselves different from one another. Studies show how they cooperate less and exhibit more competition or rivalry. DZ twins also tend to be physically more distinct than MZ twins, and it is known that appearances affect others' perceptions and reactions. Moreover, development of polarised identities can mean different interests and activities that can influence school-work, and IQ test performance.

Such effects are clearly evident in published twin correlations, even if they're brushed aside. What is being reported as 'genetic', with high heritability, can be explained by difference-making interactions between real people. In other words, parents and children are sensitive, reactive, living beings, not hollow mechanical or statistical units. The consequences are likely to pervade all twin studies. But, as ever, they can grossly mislead. For example, behaviour geneticists, using the simple agricultural model, have been unable to explain even why children in the same family are so different from one another. Furthermore, these difference-making effects are likely to increase with age. In his book *Blueprint* (and many other places), Robert Plomin makes a big deal of this, declaring it as 'one of the big findings from behavioural genetic research … genetic influences become more important as we grow older'. The findings are, however, more likely to be illusions from poor methodology and its unlikely assumptions.

In sum, there are so many unlikely assumptions and biased data interpretations entailed in twin studies as to render them unsuitable for scientific conclusion. But there is one other aspect of the research that warrants mention here.

Make-Do Data

Unfortunately, trying to describe the genetics of intelligence using the Fisher/Burt model of genetics has also encouraged a make-do research culture. As Plomin's team put it about their Twins Early Development Study: 'In-person cognitive testing of the large, geographically dispersed TEDS sample has not been feasible.' Instead, the study used a mixture of shortened forms of tests, administered by parents in the home using posted booklets, testing by telephone, and via the internet.

Other twin studies have been just as bad, if not worse, in that respect. It is no use saying that these have been 'validated' through correlation with other tests: those tests have questionable validity, too. The problem is that the less controlled the testing, the more correlations can be explained by non-cognitive factors, or other errors, and the more open they are to misinterpretation.

Adopted Children's IQs

A lesser, but still much cited, device of behaviour geneticists has been the study of adopted children. As with twin studies, the logic is beguilingly simple. It consists of comparing the IQs of adopted children with IQs of both adopted parents and their biological parents. As the theory goes, adopted children share nature with their biological parents, but nurture only with their adoptive parents, so the effects of the two can be disentangled. What a brilliant idea, you might think. Indeed, results have shown some consistency. Adopted children tend to resemble their biological parents more than their adoptive parents. The correlations are mostly very small on either side (around 0.2–0.3), and they vary from study to study and test to test. But the pattern is there.

Psychologists say they're amazed by this proof of the role of genetics. But interpretation is not so straightforward. The idealistic view of the design, based on the agricultural model, is one problem. As developmental psychologist Jacquelyne Faye Jackson put it in the journal *Child Development*, the model is 'engaging because of its simplicity. However, it is critically incomplete as a model of what actually happens in family life.'

Within families there can be many uncontrolled effects – conscious or unconscious – that lead to adoptees being treated differently from other family members. Some adoptive parents worry about the personalities, 'bloodlines', and social histories of the child's biological parents, and how that might affect them. Adoptive parents also tend to hold stronger beliefs in the influence of heredity compared with non-adoptive parents. Incredibly, in some studies, prior contact between biological and adoptive families occurred. As Sandra Scarr and colleagues put it in a 1980 article, 'Adoptive parents, knowing that there is no genetic link between them and their children, may expect less similarity and thus not pressure their children to become like their parents.' Other parents may make deliberate efforts to enhance the differences. Again, we are dealing with reactive people, in dynamic contexts, not the passive circumstances the researchers assume.

There are also many reasons why IQs between adopted children and their biological parents can correlate. One of these is that placement of children for adoption has rarely been random. From their knowledge of the biological parents, adoption agencies tend to have preconceived ideas about the future intelligence of the child, and place him or her in what they think will be a compatible family environment. There is strong evidence of such 'selective placement' in adoption studies for IQ. Even within the crude model, what is environmental is again being read as 'genetic'.

Most obviously, adopted children spend the first formative period of their lives in their biological mothers' wombs. We now know of many ways in which that experience (even stress experienced by the mother *before* pregnancy) can affect both mother and child throughout life. That includes, for example, general vitality and reactions to stress, including test-taking. In addition, there is continuing physical resemblance. Much research has shown that appearances, such as facial attractiveness or height, influence how individuals become treated by teachers and other people. The similarity between biological parents and their children in such respects may mean similar effects for their self-esteem, confidence, learning aspirations, and readiness for IQ test-taking. Again, that may lead to the (weak) correlations reported.

One pervasive finding of adoption studies is that adopted children end up actually resembling their adoptive parents in *average* IQ far more than their biological parents. Big increases of up to 15 IQ points have been reported, compared with children not adopted (and, therefore continuing in the original social class background). That is a salutary reminder of the misleading power of the correlation coefficient.

Unfortunately, adoption studies, too, have been plagued with a make-do testing culture, with a disparate assortment of tests and procedures passing for 'intelligence' tests. In one recent study, for example, there was no test available at all for the adopted children, so they simply used 'years of education' as a surrogate. Again, this is important because it opens up resulting correlations to all the uncontrolled factors mentioned above. But this is merely a brief summary of the problems with twin and adoption studies. Attempts to use the essentially agricultural model continue to this day, in full knowledge of its false assumptions. But they have reached new heights of genetic illusion with the recent DNA sequencing research.

DNA: The Genie Out of the Bottle?

In twin and adoption studies researchers cannot actually 'see' the genes whose effects they claim to be measuring. The research is based on statistical models, not direct reality. That changed when genes became identified with DNA that could be extracted from cells and analysed in the laboratory.

DNA consists of long sequences of molecules called nucleotides. They differ in that each contains one of the following chemical components: adenine (A); thymine (T); cytosine (C); and guanine (G). The sequences or strands are in pairs (the famous double-helix) such that A matches to T and C matches to G. Each gene consists of many thousands of these, with different genes comprising different sequences. The different sequences are used as templates for the assembly of different strings of amino acids.

It's those strings that make up the different proteins in cells (actually through a 'handing over' of the sequence through an intermediate, called messenger RNA).

Nearly all – at least 99 per cent – of our genes are identical from individual to individual. But occasionally one of the nucleotides in the sequence has been replaced with another. Instead of the same nucleotides at that location in the population we get a 'single nucleotide polymorphism', or SNP. Different SNPs might mean different proteins, and altered function, in different individuals, although the vast majority of these genetic variants have no known phenotypic consequence; they are 'neutral'. Nevertheless, it's those SNP differences, and their possible association with IQ differences, that have been the focus of attention (Figure 2.2). Brilliant advances in molecular biology have made it possible to describe versions of SNPs that different individuals actually have. Procedures have developed into an industrial-scale enterprise done by machines and computers at rapid speed and rapidly reducing cost. And it only requires a drop of blood or a mouth swab. This is what the Human Genome Project has been about.

Individual 1

DNA strand 1: CCGATATGCCGGTT**A**GCGCTT

DNA strand 2: GGCTATACGGCCAA**T**CGCGAA

Individual 2

DNA strand 1: CCGATATGCCGGTT**C**TGCGCTT

DNA strand 2: GGCTATACGGCCAA**G**ACGCGAA

Figure 2.2   Illustration of substitution of nucleotides across two individuals, creating an SNP (there are two strands in the DNA, one from each parent).

Immediately it occurred to behaviour geneticists that the limitations of twin and adoption studies could at last be overcome. All we have to do is measure people's IQs, get a molecular biologist to sequence for SNPs, and so discover any associations between them. The deep faith has been that this will identify 'genes for intelligence', and who does or does not have them. Again, reports were soon being laced with terms like 'exciting', 'breath-taking', and 'momentous shift', with Robert Plomin declaring the gene 'genie' to be out of the bottle. Over the last two decades dozens of such genome-wide association studies (GWAS) have been conducted, all confident that the crucial associations would be found. The old problem about correlations not being causes lurks in the background, but forgotten in the mist of excitement. Instead, you will read or hear 'linked to' quite a lot – a term both ambiguous and suggestive.

It hasn't happened, anyway. Statistically reliable correlations have been few and miniscule, and were not replicated in repeat investigations. To date, no gene or SNP has been reliably associated with the normal range even of IQ (overlooking the problem of correlations and causes, or knowing what IQ really measures). The disappointments were almost palpable, and some researchers talked of abandoning the chase. In his book *Blueprint*, Robert Plomin says, 'I pondered retirement . . . My misery about these false starts had lots of company, because many other GWA studies failed to come up with replicable results. The message slowly sank in that there are hardly any associations of large effect.'

Polygenic Scores

Then another idea emerged. Individual associations may not be evident in the way expected because they're too weak. But why not just add the strongest weak ones together until a statistically significant association with individual differences is obtained? It's a sort of 'never mind the quality, feel the width' solution. Such 'polygenic scores' have now taken over the enterprise. And some (albeit still weak) correlations with IQ scores have been reported. Perhaps the most cited study is that of James Lee and colleagues, published in the journal *Nature Genetics* in 2018. They had to use extraordinary strategies (see below), but reported polygenic score associated with around 10 per cent of the variation in 'years of education', taken as a measure of intelligence. But, it is claimed, the strategy at least showed the 'importance' of genetics for IQ. That, after all, has been the aim all along.

Again it all seems beguilingly impressive. Practical implications were soon teeming out. Robert Plomin has suggested that polygenic scores should be available from all infants at birth. They could predict possible problems in school. Never mind the 11-plus: here's the *zero*-plus exam. Other authors – in an echo of past eugenics – have proposed their use for embryo selection for intelligence.

Impressed by possibilities, the Joint Research Centre of the European Union has suggested that 'Genetic data could potentially also be of interest to employers, e.g. to screen potential job candidates and to manage career trajectories.' As they say, some laboratories already offer genetic tests to companies for such purposes. And clever marketing has seen millions of people scampering to learn their genetic horoscopes in DNA self-testing kits (crossing palms with silver in the process). So mesmerising has the story been that the flaws have been side-stepped. But all the research with GWAS/ polygenic scores involves a lot of assumptions.

Or Just Another Damp Squib?

There has been an enormous counterblast against polygenic scores as the latest in a long line of snake-oil breakthroughs. DNA expert Keith Baverstock has described them as 'fishing expeditions', looking for correlations between SNPs and complex individual differences and hoping (without any evidence whatsoever) that they are causes. To understand these issues, just bear a few figures in mind. One of the early surprises of the Human Genome Project was the number of genes that humans possess. Initially it had been assumed that proteins do most things necessary in the body, and as there are *at least* 100,000 of them, so we should have that number of genes. It turns out that we have around 20,000.

Next, consider the numbers of nucleotides that make up the genes. There are at least *three billion* of them in the human genome (actually six billion because we get a copy from each parent). The vast majority of these – about 99 per cent – are identical from person to person (that's also a measure of how genetically alike we are). On average, an SNP – the nucleotides that may vary, as in Figure 2.2 – occurs only once in every 300 nucleotides. But that means there are many *millions* of SNPs (estimates vary) in the human genome.

On the other hand, we also know that nearly all these variations are functionally neutral: it doesn't matter which version you have, they work equally well (I explain why in Chapter 3, but have a look at the NIH website). Trying to segregate these relatively few SNPs that supposedly make a difference from those that do not is difficult enough for a well-defined medical condition. But for traits as scientifically nebulous as IQ, using only statistical correlations as evidence, the enterprise seem highly naive. And there are other problems.

First, as with twin and adoption studies, the hunt for statistical associations assumes that 'effects' of SNPs are independent of one another. Estimated associations between SNPs and IQ can simply be added together to make up the polygenic scores. As mentioned in the quotes above – and explained further in Chapter 3 – such independence is now known to be highly unlikely. Interactions between the products of genes, and between those and different environments, can mean that those correlations are misleading.

Second, the correlations are still very small, and their long-term consistency unknown. So, in order to 'force' statistically significant results, investigators have had to swell study samples to include IQs – or some approximations – from hundreds of thousands of individuals. That means 'pooling' data from dozens of smaller, but highly disparate, studies under different, rough-and-ready, testing regimes. I hope you get the picture. In clouds of millions of data points of doubtful accuracy, the scope for spurious associations is enormous. In a paper entitled 'The deluge of spurious correlations in Big Data' in 2017, mathematicians Cristian Calude and Giuseppe Longo showed that arbitrary correlations in large databases are inevitable. They appear in randomly generated data due to the size of the database, not because of anything meaningful in them.

This point was amusingly illustrated in a 2020 paper by population geneticist Andrew Kern. From governmental statistics he tabulated the gross domestic products of 10 European countries plus the USA. He then computed a polygenic score for a common roadside weed that grows in all of them. He found a significant correlation between the weeds' polygenic scores and GDP. Yes – apparently the weeds' genes predict a country's GDP.

Kern illustrated how such spurious correlations are also due to what is called 'populations stratification'. In common weeds it arises (among other things) from what is called 'genetic drift'. Variations in genes (and SNPs) irrelevant to survival just randomly become more frequent in some (sub)populations than others. In humans it has become prominent for other reasons. All modern societies have arisen from centuries of immigrant streams. Different streams probably carry different sets of such (benign) SNPs. They have also tended to disperse unevenly across different social classes. But different social classes experience differences in learning opportunities, and much about the design of IQ tests, education, and so on, reflects those differences, irrespective of true abilities. Again, the scope for meaningless correlations is obvious and enormous.

Through cultural affiliations and marriage, such spurious associations can persist across many generations. A parallel is found in human surnames, which are inherited with genes. Studies of English surnames find that social class differences established in Norman times (eleventh and twelfth centuries AD) have persisted over as many as 20–30 generations. Even today, individuals bearing elite surnames from Norman and medieval times remain over-represented in the wealthier and better-educated classes in Britain. That may well mean, by the way, that your surname also predicts your IQ (and much else) without the need for hugely expensive polygenic scores.

It has become clear, in other words, that polygenic scores are prone to such distortions. And attempts to correct for them statistically are inadequate. That is evident from looking at polygenic scores within families. There, we would expect the effects of population stratification to be reduced (although not eliminated). When that is done, the small associations between polygenic scores and IQs previously reported disappear. Unsurprisingly, then, it has been found that polygenic scores for prediction of educational ability or IQ have such little predictability as to be highly questionable.

Just like IQ tests, polygenic scores may have convincing 'face' validity. But as epidemiologist Cecil Janssens pointed out in a 2019 critique in *Human Molecular Genetics*, they have no 'construct' validity. So we have the amazing spectacle of scientists using a measure of who knows what to seek (miniscule) correlations with another measure of who knows what at the cost of millions of pounds of public money.

Precision Science?

Yet again, we need to be aware of the make-do testing culture in this area. Investigators talk about 'IQ' and 'intelligence' testing. But the reality is a parody of precision science. For example, much of the recent research has used the UK Biobank, which is a dataset from about half a million participants who volunteered their blood for gene sequencing. 'Fluid intelligence' of individuals was assessed in a *two-minute*, time-limited, 13-item test. It was administered in a reception centre on a computer or on a web-based application at a later 'moment' at home (see ukbiobank.ac.uk, Category 100027). In others the pretence of testing has been abandoned altogether, and 'years of education' adopted as a surrogate for intelligence. I suspect that pet owners would not accept a measure of their dogs' intelligence so easily.

In this chapter I have tried to provide a glimpse of the methodological contortions employed in trying to sustain a particular nature–nurture picture. We have covered a lot of ground, but that reflects the determination of the intelligence gene hunters devoted to the agricultural model. Whatever they are busy with, it seems they are simply describing in obscure scientific terms the class structure of modern societies and their long histories. But the fundamental problem lies in both the nature of the gene and of intelligence. I start to elucidate them both in the next chapter.

3 Intelligent Systems

The dominant concept of intelligence is based on IQ, which is based, in turn, on the concept of the gene. Indeed IQ testing is very largely rooted in that concept. So, if I am trying to change the concept of intelligence in this book (which I am) it's obvious that we must first tackle the concept of the gene.

That's what I start to do in this chapter. Like all concept change – among academics as well as the general reader – it can be difficult, even vexing. Many have described the way that the gene has acquired God-like status in people's minds. In *The Selfish Gene*, Richard Dawkins said 'they created us body and mind', giving people the impression of an autonomous 'cognitive' agent. US President Bill Clinton described the laboratory sequencing of the human genome (the Human Genome Project) as 'learning the language in which God created life'. Many biologists still refer to the genome – the full complement of genes – as 'The Book of Life'. It is comforting (if not ironic) that Dawkins' new (2020) book is called *Outgrowing God*, which, he says (right there on the cover), 'is for anyone who wants to face up to the comforting prop of an imaginary friend'.

Those words nicely summarise my task in this chapter, though the friend I will be asking you to face up is only imaginary in how we perceive its role in intelligence, not its existence. Changing those perceptions is also difficult because there are some things about the gene that now seem self-evident and are widely accepted. Surely, you may well think, there are 'genetic' diseases, genetic susceptibilities, and 'genetic' traits. They run in families, after all. And in species. A chimp growing up in a penthouse will still grow a tail. A human developing in the trees will definitely not. 'It might be useful to be able to fly', says an article in the journal *Biomed Central*. It's impossible, it says, 'because the form of an organism is made during its embryonic development by following developmental programmes encoded in our genes'.

Well, the old model of the universe, with the sun and constellations going around the earth, was self-evident too. Hundreds of years of mounting counter-evidence were needed to overthrow it. Somewhat similarly, the whole concept of the gene has been undergoing radical revision lately. Serious reflection was compelled by even early findings of the Human Genome Project. It has been much accelerated by the disappointing results of the DNA sequencing splurge that followed. Molecular biologists have also been revealing so much more about what really goes on inside cells and organisms – including what was there at the origins of life itself.

In the Beginning

In the beginning was ... ? Well, astrophysicists are now fairly sure that the earth originated between 12 and 15 billion years ago. Most people will think of that state as anarchic, tumultuous, and disorganised; that it needed some special creative agent to harmonise things and create life. The Ancient Greeks talked about an 'ordering principle' for things in general, and 'vital spirits' and 'souls' for living things. But fairly recent advances in physics, and then biophysics, have revealed a more plausible and unifying picture.

The earth then, as since, was never a homogeneous mass of matter. It consisted, then, as now, of uneven distributions of substances and of energy. For example, heat and pressure vary enormously within and between the earth's core, crust, and atmosphere. The heat and light of the sun create other disequilibria or gradients. Those create the energy flows (light, heat, and gravity) that drive so many complex, structured activities on earth, just as water over a cliff forms waterfalls, or creates spirals around a plughole. Uneven distributions of energy tend to rebalance through the most economical means possible. In doing so, changes in matter itself, including the emergence of complex relations and structures, emerge.

Examples are legion. Familiar in the café are patterns magically appearing on coffee – duly called *latte art*. It actually consists of uneven distribution of

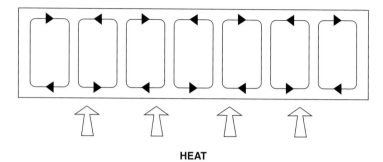

HEAT

Figure 3.1 Bénard cells forming in a layer of liquid.

espresso emulsion and microfoam milk, driven by the quick energy injection from a 'striking' rod. In the laboratory, there are many others. A layer of liquid between two plates, heated from below, can be seen to consist of closely packed convection cells moving in alternate directions (known as Bénard cells, after the person who studied them) (Figure 3.1). That emerging structure is simply the most economical way of dispersing the energy.

Even children know that the physical world is full of such ordered complexity, from ice patterns on windows to the crystals of many minerals. Other forms are patently more dynamic, like the cycles of our solar system, seasonal and daily rhythms, whorls, eddies, and currents in rivers and waterfalls, tornado vortices, and so on. When two or more entities are involved, more elaborate constructions can emerge. Some chemical reactions in the laboratory emulate *latte art* in creating distinct patterns, in different colours, and changing over long periods of time.

In all cases, the natural thermodynamics are producing *self-organisation*. In her book *Complexity*, Melanie Mitchell describes how 'large numbers of relatively simple entities organise themselves, without the benefit of any central controller, into a collective whole that creates patterns, uses information, and, in some cases, evolves and learns'. In *Understanding Evolution*, Kostas Kampourakis describes how we get design without designers. I hope you can see where we are going.

Then There Was Life . . .

Scientists are now fairly sure that life originated in such ways. Charles Darwin famously suggested that it could have arisen from chemical reactions, 'in some warm little pond, with all sorts of ammonia and phosphoric salts, light, heat, electricity, etc. present'. And maybe, he went on, 'a protein compound was chemically formed, ready to undergo still more complex changes . . .'. That may not have been too far from the truth (proteins often being described as the main constituents, or 'building blocks', of life).

Biochemists have played with 'primordial soups' in the laboratory in various ways. In some experiments, electrical discharges passed through mixtures of hydrogen, methane, ammonia, and water vapour have produced a variety of amino acids, themselves the constituents of proteins, and other organic molecules. Others have employed the catalytic (reaction boosting) properties of metals, such as iron and nickel, abundant on the floors of hot, acidic oceans, along with hydrogen and carbon gases. '[W]e observed 29 metabolism-like chemical reactions, including those that produce some of the essential chemicals of metabolism, for example precursors to the building blocks of proteins or RNA', said Cambridge scientist Markus Ralser in a Wellcome Trust interview in 2014. RNA (ribonucleic acid) is thought to have been a possible bearer of 'genetic' information before DNA arrived.

Natural processes could even have wrapped these metabolising mixtures inside fatty membranes. As Bruce Damer put it in a blog post,

> As the pools dried down, they became surrounded by a glistening bathtub ring composed of layered membranous structures formed by fatty acids delivered by the meteoritic material. Between those silvery drying layers, the organic building blocks of amino acids and nucleic acids jostled into position. The first primitive biopolymers were forming, and our origin of life story is now beginning.

Either way, not only can amino acids so form, they can also readily combine into strings (polymers), the basic structures of peptides and proteins. They have 'autocatalytic' properties, meaning they can foster or speed up other chemical reactions, including those boosting their own production. Polymer strings then created extensive reactive networks. This may have constituted primordial metabolisms: self-sustaining, self-organising systems, absorbing energy from their surroundings to maintain their structures, and dissipating wastes back into the environment. Such 'autocatalytic sets' have been well demonstrated in laboratories.

In the mix would have been small molecules called nucleic acids. These can also spontaneously polymerise into strings of RNA and DNA. It has been realised that, probably before a later role as memory molecules or genes, RNAs could catalyse the formation of amino acid strings to form peptides and proteins. Even dilute mixtures could thus form interacting ensembles with life-like attributes, without genes as such.

They Became Systems

These assortments of aliens got along together because doing so main-tained their integrity over continual environmental change, at least for a period of time. That is what most distinguished them from non-living molecular mixtures. While some components are being stressed, others are adjusting their reactions to compensate. They became 'systems'. The reac-tion properties of molecules generally, after all, are not those of rigid stimulus–response elements. Their reactions are modifiable, depending on physical or chemical contexts (e.g. temperature, pH), and even the products of their own reactions. That is basic chemistry. Interactions between chemicals in a mixture, such as to compensate for some disturb-ance, are also well known in the laboratory. That's what things like the 'stabilising agents' you can see in the list of ingredients are for in many processed foods.

Imagine a change in the surrounding environment, such as a decrease in pH (an increase in acidity). That changes the three-dimensional shape of a particular protein in the mix, which is important for assisting energy flows. Now consider that the result of *that* change is to change the shape of another protein. And the result of *that*, finally, is to nullify the effect of the rise in pH (either by increasing the flow of energy in some other way, or a reaction that increases alkalinity). That system is more likely to survive the change. It will be 'naturally selected'. So the components become 'bonded' as a system of mutual dependence in that sense.

Go one step further. Imagine the fall of pH is usually followed by the incursion of some toxic chemical. The fall of pH changes the shape of a protein as before, and changes the shape of another. But the effect of that second change is to nullify the effects of the toxin *before it can permeate the system*. Now we have an 'anticipatory system' predicting a future change from something happening now. This is like basic association learning: dogs salivating when they hear the bell that predicts the meal to follow. It is still only natural responses to energy gradients, but that, too, will be more likely to survive as an integral system. It will be naturally selected.

Chemists and biochemists have been exploring and tinkering with such networks for many years. The theoretical biologist Robert Rosen, in the 1970s, offered a rigorous mathematical treatise on such 'anticipatory systems'. Properties emerge from relations in networks that transcend those of independent components. More recently, systems scientist Simon McGregor and colleagues used computer models of chemical networks to describe associative learning in a diversity of remarkably simple and plausible chemical solutions.

Molecular networks with anticipatory properties are regularly being reported in cells today. Biochemists sometimes refer to them as tuneable 'molecular grammars', by analogy with human language, where the rules of grammar can generate an infinite number of novel utterances. I have referred to them as 'Biogrammars'. The rules can be thought of as associations dependent upon other variables or other associations (often in huge numbers), just as in ordinary speech the same sound can predict different things in different contexts. Finally, in those first systems, as components reproduced and accumulated, they may have frequently split. That's a kind of reproduction by division (binary fission) seen in single-cell organisms today. And new ensembles would be constantly forming. That, at least, would have been some sort of life.

Intelligent Life

The important thing is that these primitive systems were able to maintain integrity across changing environments because components could cooperate, mutually compensate for each other, and acquire, or 'learn', new compensations in the process.

That's intelligence; and it was there from the beginning. The 'beginning' (of life) could not have happened without it. Intelligent systems have been a powerful force in the fountain of evolution as anticipatory systems. Of course, simpler systems would have coalesced, adding further components and energy efficiency. So take one step further, and add to the primordial cell surface special receptor molecules acutely sensitive to environmental changes. Then add other molecular components that endow the system with movement. Now its energy fuel, and other resources, can be pro-actively sought, rather than passively awaited. That intelligence even appears to have endowed the cell with 'agency'. But it derives from physico-chemical realities, not supernatural forces. It all helps explain the astonishing – almost unbelievable – complexities that followed, as I hope to show.

An important theme is that environments that change rapidly over time, involving more factors, can reach higher scales of complexity. Much of the rest of this book is about the different levels of intelligent systems that emerged and evolved in order to survive complex environmental changes. Each level or stage can be thought of as collaboration between components, involving reconfiguration of relations between them. Like learning new rules of engagement, this fostered assimilation of deeper environmental patterns, and thus greater predictability and survival within them.

In the meantime, that gives us not just a definition, but, more importantly, a functional *characterisation* of intelligence. Intelligence is sensitivity to change that depends on other changes. The dependencies may be simple correlations between two variables, which I talked about in Chapter 1. That is information for anticipation or predictability: light at dawn predicts impending rise in temperature, and so on. More realistically, even in primitive molecular soups, the dependencies will go much deeper, between multitudes of variables, in deep three-dimensional networks, in patterns that change over time. A chemical reaction may depend on pH, which depends on salinity, which depends on temperature, which depends on time of day; and so on. There will be long chains and levels of correlational patterns in most real-world systems, especially as they are changing with time. Three dimensions thus become four, and the correlation patterns are more akin to a movie than a photograph.

In real life, too, such co-variations may well be non-linear. That is, steps in one are bigger or smaller than steps in the other(s), giving rise to further complexity. But it's been shown that any living system that can register those chains and levels can respond creatively and fruitfully. It will be a 'dynamic system', able to make more precise predictions and inform its behaviour. Uncertain futures can be tracked. It will be very intelligent. A fundamental message, then, is that intelligence is to be found in relations between components, not in the components themselves. I will be repeating that message many times.

The Environment

In passing, this also tells us more about natural environments. Many scientists still cling to an agricultural view of the environment: independent factors that help or hinder some specific aspect of living things and their development and survival. In fact, it is such correlational *patterns* that we, and all living things, are swimming in all the time and that are most important to survival. That's one reason we have failed to perceive and describe the environment properly. We can just about imagine, or visualise, three or four variables mutually dependent in that way. We may even describe them verbally: the bus is usually on time, except in rush hour, especially on Fridays (and so on). Beyond that, the complexity defies verbal description, although we may have a hunch or gut-feeling about it.

Scientists have dealt with that problem through the language of mathematics. Information theorists have come up with a range of measures of complex patterns – basically ones that quantify how much change in one variable can predict change in one or more others. The advent of the digital computer has greatly facilitated this. It's what mathematical modelling, as in artificial intelligence or the current COVID-19 epidemic is about: looking for correlational patterns and extrapolating from them to predict the future.

By using such information, living things don't just change their 'state' in response to certain conditions; they also change the 'rules' by which they do so. This is reminiscent of the theory of intelligence of the great developmental psychologist Jean Piaget. He said that animals become intelligent through a dual process of assimilation (of experience) and accommodation (of the intelligent system) to allow increasing levels of predictability in the world. We are now in a better position to understand how all that was present in those primitive molecular networks. *But there were still no genes.*

Why No Genes?

There were still no genes, at least as popularly conceived. The strings of RNA, and then DNA, probably arrived on the scene, as what we now call genes, much later, and it's important to understand why. The original molecular networks faced highly changeable circumstances, not merely gently fluctuating, ebb-and-flow conditions. Much was going on rapidly, multi-dimensionally, and irreversibly. If ensembles of proteins, nucleotides, sugars, fats, and other molecules persisted – as they seem to have done – it could only be because they could mutually adjust to those constant changes.

What it is important to grasp is that fixed genetic information cannot do that. The popularly conceived DNA template can only yield a fixed copy of itself. It can only 'code' for the same proteins, on a recurring basis, in fairly constant environments. In modern neo-Darwinian theory, the genetic templates have been arrived at through natural selection of random mutations – through 'survival of the fittest', as the cliché goes. That has been important in evolution, in helping organisms to 'adapt' to parts of the environment. But, like the clothing manufacturer still trying to sell yesterday's fashions, it has its limitations. Logically, genetic selection is only possible so long as the same environment remains steady across generations while the selected genes get passed on. In chapter four of *Origin of Species*, Darwin himself acknowledged that 'natural selection generally acts with extreme slowness'. But, as we have just seen, for the continual everyday struggle with more complex environments, systems more *intelligent* than that would have been favoured as means of survival.

Genes, that is, became extremely useful in relation to fairly constant aspects of environments. Nuts and bolts are always needed, even when the machines and parts they are used in change over time. In cells, genes are reliable sources of cell components, available as and when needed, across generations. More changeable environments demand self-organised intelligent systems for survival.

We've Had It All Wrong

This is a radical, even revolutionary view. It inverts the conventional picture of the relation between gene and organism. But it is one being forced upon us through the failures of genetics described in the previous chapter. Decades of entrenched dogma have told us that the genes are the activists. Cells and organisms, and all they do, are merely passive instruction-bearers in the command line. Now, it seems, things are the other way around. Failing to understand that explains why we've failed to understand intelligence in general.

This point is now being made by many others. In a paper in the journal *BioEssays* in 1990, evolutionary biologist Frederik Nijhout criticised the metaphor of genes as 'controlling', or as 'programmes for', development. Studies in 2019 by Benoit Pujol and colleagues have shown that in the wild – that is, outside the unreal conditions of the laboratory or breeding station – natural selection of genes is subordinate to other adaptable processes. Physiologist Denis Noble put it well in an interview with Suzan Mazur in *Huff Post Science* (22 November 2015):

> The modern synthesis has got causality in biology wrong. Genes, after all, if they're defined as DNA sequences, are purely passive. DNA on its own does absolutely nothing until activated by the rest of the system . . . DNA is not a cause in an active sense. I think it is better described as a passive data base which is used by the organism to enable it to make the proteins that it requires.

In sum, genes are merely templates for copying a sequence from one string of molecules to another. As Keith Baverstock explains: 'Although vital information derives from genes, these are in some senses like the merchants that provide the materials out of which a house is built: they don't design the house or build it, but without them the house can't be built.'

The rest of this chapter illustrates how the whole operates as a dynamic intelligent system.

Sensing Change

The cell as we know it today has thousands of different components, many organised in separate compartments also enclosed in membranes. Far from being dumb microscopic blobs, cells are exquisitely sensitive to changes (stimuli) in the surrounding milieu, and use patterns in the changes to create intelligence about how to respond.

That starts at the outer surface. Many years ago, biologists discovered the surface membrane to be studded with special molecules serving as receptors. These are acutely sensitive to a wide range of stimuli in the surrounding environment: nutrients, salts, toxins, and so on, as well as physical bumps and shocks. Until recently it was assumed that the membrane receptors acted independently of each other, stimulus–response style, each just mechanically passing on a GO–STOP signal to the inside. That turns out to be far from the case. The outside environment is raining constant stimulus storms onto the membranes. The receptors are extremely good at picking up the ever-changing correlation patterns in those storms. They do this by 'talking' to each other, much like the molecular networks described above.

The bacterium *E.coli*, for example, survives in liquid media in many places, including the human body. It swims around using its multi-strand tails (flagella) until its surface receptors detect the presence of a nutrient such as glucose. The bacterium needs to get to the source; but the signal will usually be diffusing through the medium from some novel direction and distance from the cell. How can the bacterium home in on it?

Intuitively, a simple cue–response function might seem like the answer: simply turn to the signal and swim towards it. However, that's more difficult than it seems. The cell cannot 'see', after all. Like a storm of pebbles thrown at your front door, independent 'hits' of nutrient molecules on the curved surface of the cell give no precise indication of which direction they came from.

However, because of the curved surface, hits from a given direction will be spread out in a specific space–time pattern correlating with that direction

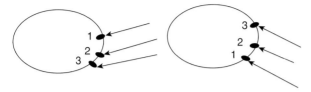

Figure 3.2 Nutrient direction signalled by space–time correlation on cell receptors (1, 2, 3 signifying the order of reception).

(Figure 3.2). The pattern itself changes as the cell itself moves. But, by registering the correlation pattern, the cell can predict the original location. It happens in an amazing sequence of steps described by biologist John Parkinson and colleagues (as well as other teams), involving interactions between receptors and several other components. The end result is to send not a simple signal, but an equivalent correlation pattern to the interior of the cell. The signal sets its flagella moving in the correct combination. But the important thing is that all cells must do this kind of assimilation of environmental structure. It has even led to cell membranes being referred to as 'little brains'. There is no overall programme or conductor of these affairs, only the time-and-motion intelligence registering the ever-changing patterns around them.

Networks, Loops, and Tunes

Clever as all that may seem, it's only opinion-forming chatter at the doorway compared with what happens next, when the opinion is passed on. Inside the cell are other networks of almost unbelievable scale, even in yeasts and bacteria. Their role is not that of 'mindless biochemical machines', as Kevin Mitchell called them. Their function is to extract further patterns from that initial 'opinion'. It does *that* by comparing what is being said from one set of receptors with what is being said from others, so detecting deeper patterns among them. In that way, further intelligence is gained, further changes are anticipated, and the best next response is more accurately predicted.

Those pathways can involve hundreds or thousands of components, in cascades of signals. As with the molecular ensembles described above, the 'messages' are not simple STOP–GO signals. They are spread out, space–time patterns, like the echo-locations used by a bat, changing rapidly over time, and predicting a likely sequence of events. Even partial or fleeting inputs can thus be extrapolated into more meaningful messages, rather as you can usually make sense of a garbled word or sentence in speech from its wider context.

A prominent feature of these networks is the presence, in large numbers, of feed-forward and feedback loops. Such loops are very important for enhancing intelligence-gathering in the cell, but they have also been vital in the evolution of 'higher' forms, including human intelligence. So we should dwell on them a little. *Feed-forward* consists of a signal passed from one part of a system to another, informing a reaction. When someone throws a ball at you a feed-forward signal from the brain informs your hand where the ball will be in a few milliseconds' time. Frost on the window induces you to put on extra clothing before going outside on a cold day. A 'green' at traffic lights gets a car to move off.

Feedback is when the result of the reaction proceeds backwards to (possibly) change or modulate the original signal. It may be positive or negative in effect. When you get outside and find it's not so cold after all, you take a layer off. Other traffic on the road may advise changing a green light to red. A rising room temperature switches off the signal from the room thermostat to the boiler or heater. In sum, feed-forward sends a signal, but feedback, sensitive to wider contexts of information, may modify it. The result is more intelligence and greater precision in operation (Figure 3.3).

Such feed-forward/feedback loops are a ubiquitous device in the intelligent activities of living things at all levels, including physiology, brains, and human social activities – which are covered much more in later chapters. (I will occasionally refer to FF/FB loops, or bottom-up, top-down systems). The important point is that layers of such loops 'nest' sideways and upwards into hierarchies sensitive to deeper patterns, in the way that letters are nested in words nested in sentences. By using such loops, the networks are being continuously reconfigured in response to experiences. That is, the networks 'learn' and modify responses accordingly. This is a powerfully adaptable way of bringing previous experience to bear on current – often fuzzy, imperfect, or novel – inputs.

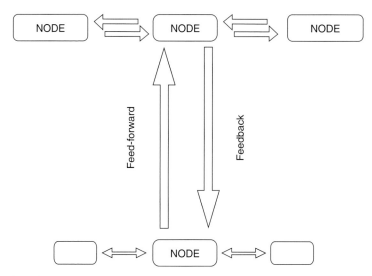

Figure 3.3 Feed-forward/feedback loop. Nodes are subgroups of signalling molecules or other cell components.

Understanding such loops has transformed how cell biologists think of the cell. In the past, we have tended to think of cell processes as mechanical, automatic, and independent of each other. But the language most prominent today is that of cooperation, democracy, teamwork, adaptability, and even cognition. 'Can cells think?' was the title of one paper in the journal *Cellular and Molecular Life Sciences*. The self-organised order has even attracted musical metaphors like 'orchestration', 'symphony', 'the signaling ballet', or the 'Dance to the Tune of Life' (the title of Denis Noble's 2016 book). It has given rise to a new field of 'cognitive biology', duly recognising the cell as an intelligent system.

Intelligent Behaviour

Unsurprisingly, those investigating the intelligence of the cell have regularly been stumped by the sheer complexity and dynamics of the networks. Descriptions of even the simplest of these can sound quite arcane. The patterns are so abstract that they can only be revealed through statistical modelling in computers with dense mathematics. However, explicit evidence of intelligent processing is there in observable behaviours, even in relatively simple organisms. 'Learning and memory – abilities associated with a brain or, at the very least, neuronal activity – have been observed in protoplasmic slime, a unicellular organism with multiple nuclei.' So says science writer Philip Ball, with a hint of incredulity, in an article in the journal *Nature* in 2008.

Paramecium is a single-cell pond organism, that normally swims towards light. In one experiment, light at one end of a container was associated with a mild electric current. The *Paramecium* soon learned to avoid the light and swim for the dark. In the reverse conditions they did the opposite. They were obviously learning to use the correlational pattern to predict change in one variable from values in another. Similarly with *E.coli* studied by Ilias Tagkopoulos and colleagues: they found that this single cell could learn an association between temperature change *now* and oxygen levels a little later. That's the kind of change experienced when the bug gets into your mouth and then swallowed into your gut. The association is such that the bug anticipates the drop in oxygen levels and rapidly recruits alternative (anaerobic, not requiring oxygen) metabolic networks before it gets there.

As biologists Amit Mitchell and Yitzhak Pilpel explain in a review in 2011, 'A diversity of microorganisms, including *Escherichia coli*, *Vibrio cholerae*, and several yeast species, were shown to use a predictive regulation strategy that uses the appearance of one stimulus as a cue for the likely arrival of a subsequent one.' A burgeoning literature has also been reporting such strategies even in plants. Such findings have given rise to a whole new field of 'cognitive biology'. Today's molecular biologists are reporting 'intelligence' in bacteria, 'cognitive resources' in single cells, 'bio-information intelligence', 'cell intelligence', 'metabolic memory', and 'cell knowledge' – all terms appearing in recent literature.

How Genes Are (Intelligently) Used

Although torrents of DNA-hype have induced us to think of the genes as recipes or programmes for making an organism, the metaphors are misleading. They imply a kind of conscious agency that the genes do not have. We may think of them as recipes for *ingredients*, to be then used as resources. But they do not do the gathering, the preparations, cooking and icing, nor decide how the same ingredients can be used for many different recipes. Genes do not have the predictability, the tools, skills, and sheer *nous* for inventing the recipe in the first place. The idea that dumb chemical sequences constitute, on their own, sets of instructions for making 'all that we are' (Robert Plomin) or contain 'a program for making a human being with typical human nature' (Kevin Mitchell) is flimsy when we come to think of it.

The genes come in as servants to intelligent systems, not their directors. Cells have to do many different things: grow, divide, specialise, stream energy, produce hormones, renew cell receptors, signal to other cells, and so on. Often the dynamics will 'call' for ingredients – RNAs, peptides, enzymes, other proteins – from the genes. That's what the genes are there for, to provide ingredients when required. They do nothing without instructions from the cell as a whole, then always in carefully controlled steps contingent on numerous other factors. I cannot give a comprehensive picture of all that here. A brief summary of the cascades of signals and interactions will have to suffice.

The first step in using genes is for cell signals to penetrate the chromosomes and unwind the spools of proteins around, and interacting with, the DNA strands. Other signals then activate a number of key mediators on the DNA strand, called transcription factors (TFs). These TFs in turn operate through a variety of other components with self-explanatory titles like promoters, enhancers, co-activators, and co-regulators. These all form a cooperative team, orchestrated by intra- and extracellular signalling patterns.

Correspondingly, the genes are not simple 'switches'. They have evolved with flanking regions on the DNA strands, sensitive to these regulatory factors. Like the layers of identity checks to your online banking accounts (username, password, date of birth, and so on), those factors operate in different combinations to further regulate payout (called transcription). The combination governs whether transcription will occur at all, and with how much product (Figure 3.4).

Transcription from gene to product is rarely direct, though. The DNA sequence of components (the nucleotides) is first copied into

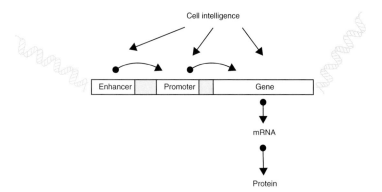

Figure 3.4   Gene transcription depends on cell intelligence.

a complementary sequence of similar nucleotides on 'messenger' RNA (mRNA). This mRNA carries the sequence out of the nucleus, into the wider cell. It then serves as the template for bringing amino acids into line to form peptides and proteins, using a range of enzymes.

And that's where cell intelligence figures again. The old, standard picture is one in which the gene sequence 'codes' for the sequence of amino acids to make up one – and only one – protein:

One gene → one mRNA → one protein.

According to that picture, the proteins then (somehow) get together to form a 'genetic programme'. Chance variation in genes from individual to individual (be they bacteria or people) results in accidentally different programmes, so the story goes. Then, with some variation from the environment, plus random effects (or 'noise'), different programmes make individual differences in traits. Perhaps it's hardly surprising that authors like Murray, Plomin, Haier, and Mitchell have presented it as a picture of differences in human intelligence. But we now know it's a travesty of what actually happens: that the model is far from the reality. Here's just a few – and I emphasise, a *few* – illustrations of that reality.

Strange Codes: Impossible Programmes

In fact, only 1–2 per cent of DNA is involved in making the RNA that helps make proteins. The rest transcribes as other forms of RNA involved in a vast range of other functions. As regards those genes that *do* code for proteins, the 'gene-as-instruction' point of view is still very popular. *But there is no consistent instruction.* Imagine an instruction as a long string of words. Then somebody cuts out from the sequence combinations of words that make up sentences – but *different* sentences at different times. What kind of instruction is that?

The production of messenger RNA, the first transcript from those genes, is something like that. Parts of its sequence, called *exons*, do serve as parts of protein templates. But they are interspersed with 'noncoding' fragments that are silent (are not transcribed), called *introns*. Cell processes remove the introns to bring the exons together. That process has been called RNA splicing. However, it has also been discovered that the splicing can be such as to produce different permutations of exons. That's called alternative splicing (Figure 3.5).

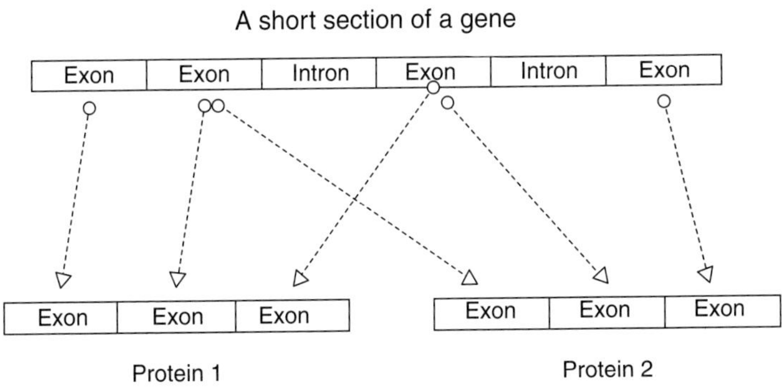

A short section of a gene

Figure 3.5   Messenger RNA is spliced, but then different exons can be brought together in different ways corresponding with different proteins from the same gene (alternative splicing).

The obvious consequence is that many different proteins can be produced *from the same gene*, with potentially widely different functions:

one gene → many proteins.

There is no consistent genetic message, instruction, or programme. Rather, the message varies under the control of the cell as a whole. We now know that this 'exon shuffling' affects the vast majority of such messages. In a 2014 paper in *Nature*, geneticist James B. Brown and colleagues reported that even in a fruit fly, one particular set of genes has the potential to encode *thousands* of different transcripts.

This picture has been confirmed by researchers analysing the actual contents of cells. In a car factory, with fixed blueprints and programmes, you would expect to see identifiable parts being assembled into identifiable vehicles. In the cell there is little correspondence between cell contents, such as peptides and proteins, and its DNA sequences. In a study in 2019, Mehran Piran and colleagues found that simply enumerating the immediate products of genes in a cell does not allow us to predict cell behaviour. Likewise, Chengran Yang and co-researchers in 2020 found little correspondence between the proteins 'in' the cell and actual gene sequences. Even genetically identical cells exhibit wide variation in their molecular networks due to different experiences. It looks as if the 'programme' arises in the cell itself, and is not prefigured in the genes at all.

More strikingly, there are a number of processes through which the intelligent cell can even change the genetic information itself. James Shapiro calls it *natural genetic engineering* (NGE) and says, in a paper in *Physics of Life Reviews*, that 'the standard model of a "Read-Only" tape that feeds instructions to the rest of the cell about individual characters [is a] dangerous oversimplification'. Now, he says, 'we have to reconsider the genome as a "read–write" (RW) information storage system'.

It's surely time to give up the idea of fixed codes or programmes in the genes. Instead we must focus on context-sensitive intelligent systems in the cell as a whole. Other facts also indicate this. There is no relation between numbers of genes and the complexity of organisms. Humans have about 20,000 genes. That's about the same as the pond-dwelling *Hydra*, and half as many as a cabbage or a carrot. And we share 99 per cent of our genes with chimpanzees and 95 per cent with mice. Rather, most of the evolution of complexity is explained by a vast expansion of signalling and metabolic networks. That includes increasing numbers of TFs, enhancers, promoters, and other regulatory elements – and, of course, more context-sensitive feed-forward/feedback loops. In these intelligent systems, programmes are constructed 'on the hoof'. Their adaptability is just what's needed in changing environments.

Heritability Futility

This brief glimpse at the intelligent biology of the cell also exposes another reality. Within any particular species, for complex traits, important for every-day function, there is little association between genetic variation and out-come variation. The intelligence of the cell takes care of that.

This has been demonstrated many times in the laboratory. For example, within a particular species, individual cells or organisms with identical genes can develop widely different traits, as needed according to circumstances. Conversely, those with different genes can develop identical traits, again as circumstances demand. Except for the few exceptional cases, it is impossible to predict the phenotype from the genotype. I will be saying more about this in Chapter 5, on the subject of development.

Of course, genes provide important resources. As with environmental defi-ciencies, their absence (as in mutations of the DNA) can be a threat to the function of cells and organisms. However, for functions crucial to survival the threat can usually be nullified by network adjustments or creation of alterna-tive pathways. Only in rare cases will associations between gene variants and outcomes be evident. Those are cases where, for example, the system cannot cope with the absence of resources, either genetic or environmental (and more about that in later chapters).

That further brings into perspective the problems with heritability estimates for intelligence in humans. First, it has become increasingly clear that intelli-gence is not a mechanical function that varies across individuals in terms of unitary strength or power. Nor can that variation simply be attributed to variation in genetic and/or environmental elements that simply add together. Those are the assumptions underlying the heritability estimates for human intelligence mentioned in Chapter 2. We now know that neither genes nor their SNPs 'act', or make differences, as independent units – a vital assumption in the twin, adoption, and gene-sequencing studies. Their effects on differences are not simply sums of their independent effects. Even at the level of the cell, we have deeply interactive intelligent systems, not mechanical programmes. Variation in complex functions is due to interactions at many levels.

Of course, there are prominent (and visible) cases where effects of different genetic resources remain. They have survived natural selection because they only relate to traits that are not important to survival. That's part of the logic of natural selection in Darwin's theory. Heritability may be high for some (usually unimportant) traits, and nullified for others that are more important to survival. And this is what has been found many times in populations of organisms in the wild. The heritabilities listed in Table 3.1, for example, were estimated not by fallible twin studies using rough-and-ready measures and unlikely statistical models. They come from well-controlled estimates in the house martin carried out by Philippe Christe and colleagues. As you can see, these heritabilities of important survival traits are miniscule compared with those (0.5–0.8) typically reported for human intelligence derived from twin studies.

Statistician Peter Schönemann sarcastically warned that heritability estimates for IQ of 60 per cent or more 'surpass anything found in the animal kingdom'.

Trait	Heritability
Wing length	0.156
Tarsus length	0.079
Body mass	0
Immunoglobulins	0.051
T-cell response	0.007
Leukocytes	0.059

Table 3.1   Heritabilities for traits important for survival in the house martin. The tarsus is a prominent foot bone. Other traits are crucial to the immune system.

It is strange that so few scholars studying the 'genetics' of intelligence have noted that. Instead, they have been lured into agricultural models of intelligent systems that are totally inappropriate. It was illustrated perfectly in the *Annual Review of Psychology* by K. Paige Harden in 2021, who still thinks that a 'directly measured' genome can reveal 'how genes and environments combine to create unique human lives'. This only ensures psychology's detention in a Dark Age.

4 Intelligence Evolving

Charles Darwin's *On the Origin of Species* is a delightfully sophisticated account of evolution. But the core ideas are not that difficult to understand. Variations in traits in individuals arise by chance, due to what we now think of as mutations in genes. Some of those trait variations are functionally better adapted to part of the environment than others. Individuals so advantaged will tend to survive and leave more offspring. Accordingly, the advantage, and the frequency of the genes causing it, will increase from generation to generation. Conversely, genes causing less advantageous or harmful variations will decrease in frequency. That is natural selection.

In *Understanding Evolution*, Kostas Kampourakis describes not only the evidence for evolution, but also the painstaking way in which investigators have pieced together ancestral trees. All that has given us huge insights into biology, generally, and human origins in particular. Many, if not most, people today accept that organisms have descended from a common ancestor through natural processes, producing new life forms from pre-existing ones.

Traditionally that has meant focusing on the more visible, tractable aspects of living things; those clearly well adapted to some aspect of the conditions in which they live. These have included body forms and appendages, obvious physiologies (such as energy sources and forms of respiration), or those stereotyped behaviours usually called 'instincts'. This accounts for the tendency to define species and groups predominantly by their morphologies and overt habits. It also presupposes that the environments to which they are well adapted will be fairly constant across generations. Without a stable criterion, there could be no consistent selection.

In Chapter 3 I drew attention to the more rapid changeability of many, if not most, aspects of natural environments. As ecologist Richard Levins explained in *Evolution in Changing Environments*, 'When our emphasis shifts to variable environments entirely new problems arise.' Therein may lie the key to understanding even more important characteristics of living things, like intelligence, and an even more thrilling evolutionary story. When the rules of the game are constantly changing, only those organisms that can keep up in a different way can survive. The point of intelligent systems is that they engender fantastic varieties of form as active, anticipatory processes. That means variation that could not arise through slow, plodding selection of genetic mutations.

Change and Complexity

The idea also helps us to understand another problem: why and how, in the course of evolution, increasingly complex forms have appeared. It was a problem that haunted Darwin. His theory could not easily account for it. In a letter to Charles Lyell, he said that it seemed impossible to answer the question, 'how did any complications of organisms profit them?'. More complex form, after all, is more difficult to develop and maintain, and more prone to catastrophic breakdown. Its selection would need to be accompanied by other advantages. Darwin, like others since, suggested that greater coordination of greater numbers of parts provides greater 'efficiency'. However, merely gathering together parts in greater numbers does not automatically explain complexity (nor, necessarily, efficiency). Where does the 'coordination' come from? As with the origin of genes, some system of coordination needs to be there *first*.

In this chapter I will be describing how intelligent systems have formed, not merely a ferment of useful variation, but also a fountain of complexity in the course of evolution. In Chapter 5 I will describe how those systems also define development, including how they utilise genes. That will include the questions of what we can mean by 'genetic causes', as in some diseases and conditions, or some obvious trait differences like eye colour. But my overall theme will be that intelligent systems, though not as visible as legs, wings, fins, or whatever, have formed a most important strand in the evolution of organisms. From their origins in molecular ensembles, in already difficult circumstances, intelligent systems underpinned survival and expansion in many different habitats.

Because intelligent systems constantly change themselves, they form a deeper engine of evolution. As the 'simpler ways of life' became filled (to use Darwin's phrase), simpler organisms were pushed out into more challenging, changeable, and less predictable environments. Only more complex adaptable forms could survive. They, in turn, filled the spaces they could, changing and making them more complex in the process – and so on, into a virtuous spiral of functions. I have already described the molecular networks that furnished adaptability and learning in single cells, even in the humble *E.coli*. In this chapter I want to illustrate how intelligent systems formed the basis of the evolution of increasingly higher levels of complexity.

Cells Get Together

Turmoil and uncertainty in changeable environments have been life's constant counterpart. Quite early in evolution it happened that living things better survived when they behaved as a team. Soon after their evolution, single cells found ways to cooperate. It made responses and behaviours possible that would be difficult for isolated individuals. Dealing with patchy or uneven supplies of food sources may have been one advantage. Being able to feed on larger prey could have been another. Resistance to predators may also have counted. Either way, single cells already had crucial preadaptations: the intelligent systems within cells were already able to register patterns from the outside environment, anticipate changes, and shape adaptable responses. They were perfectly prepared for a chemical 'dialogue' and mutual accommodation *between* cells.

The classic example, still around today, is the slime mould *Dictyostelium*, an amoeba that creeps around in soil looking for bacteria to eat, and reproducing by binary fission (Figure 4.1). When food supplies start to run out, numbers of them aggregate to form a multicellular 'slug' that slithers its way to a local high point. About 20 per cent of the cells then differentiate to form the stalk of a fruiting body that lifts most of the others into the air. These non-stalk cells

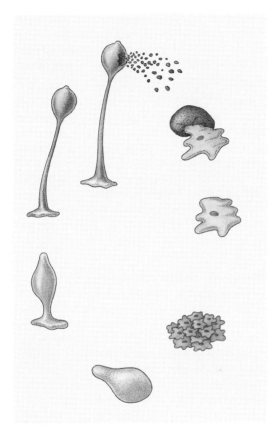

Figure 4.1   Slime mould in the process of aggregation and forming a fruiting body (Dorling Kindersley/Getty Images).

turn into dormant, resistant spores that are eventually released into the air. The wind then carries them to new locations, establishing new populations.

There are many other examples. Some are notable for forming biofilms on water surfaces, or even predatory swarms to hunt bacteria. Their intelligence also makes them opportunistic. In the wild, *Pseudomonas* species are vigorous, fast-swimming bacteria. Inside humans, some cause infections in the urinary tract, respiratory system, skin, soft tissues, bones and joints, gut, and blood. Under challenge from the immune system they also come together to form biofilms, a kind of a mucoid slime, for protection.

In all such cases, the process of aggregating is like the lone hunters' response in the forest to the scent of campfires. The 'smoke' consists of the mutual secretion of small signalling molecules, called auto-inducers. Coordination through these is called *quorum sensing* (QS). As broadcast signals, they will be hitting different individuals from different directions with different intensities. Only by detecting correlations as intensities change over direction and time (rather as you sniff around when a smoke alarm sounds) can the most likely centre of convergence be computed, and movement coordinated. For such reasons, QS is sometimes described as the 'language' of microorganisms. It forms interacting feed-forward/feedback loops coordinating millions of cells adapting to environmental changes.

What goes on between cells coordinates not merely movement, but also extensive structural and biochemical changes *within* them. It involves wholesale reconfiguration of their metabolic networks. The emergence of a new intelligent system on a new level is being witnessed. With it, other amazing powers seem to emerge. For example, laboratory experiments report colonies learning the route through a maze in order to reach food sources. As Oné R. Pagán explained in a 2019 article, 'The notion of "proto-brains" formed by individual bacterial or amoeboid cells is something that was unthinkable until very recently. Slime moulds are currently studied in terms of their "proto-cognitive" abilities.'

In such ways, from such humble beginnings, intelligence came to dominate the evolution of living things, fostering the many wonderful forms and variations we treasure. That process of emergence helps us to understand the great leaps we see in evolution, including that very special leap to human intelligence, to be described in Chapter 7.

Multicellular Systems

Whereas slime moulds had previously independent histories, true multicellular organisms originated as clones of a single cell. Following cell division the daughter cells remain attached to one another, and they will have identical genomes. But they display amazing varieties of specialised forms and behaviours, and have vastly enhanced versatility in changing environments. Not surprisingly, the leap from simple unicellularity to complex multicellularity used to be described as one of life's mysteries. The mystery is not solved, however, by looking for specific components or new genetic programmes. Rather, the transition occurred through the emergence of further intelligent systems from what had already evolved.

There is still disagreement about when it occurred; estimates range from 600 million to 2 billion years ago. And it may have occurred several times independently. However, a plausible story is that it originated from the division of single cells, the products of which continued to (literally) stick together to share their assets and cooperate. It comes with obvious costs. Compared with single cells, multicellular organisms are more difficult to form, are more vulnerable to fatal breakdown, and need more complicated nutrient delivery systems, waste dispersal systems, and so on. Reproduction is also more difficult than simple binary fission. Yet the advantages obviously outweigh those challenges. Just getting bigger helps to avoid former predators. More importantly, a wider range of functions can be coordinated, the better to deal with rapidly changing environments and more complex habitats and lifestyles. Single-celled organisms, even those that occasionally aggregate, continue to exist in comparatively narrow or specialised environments. Multicellular organisms have found adaptability in all the difficult corners and unpredictable circumstances on earth.

All of this occurs through the emergence of communication systems between the cells. In cooperating, two or more dynamical systems become 'coupled', such that the state of one is a function of the state of the other. Divisions of labour are established, and biochemical behaviours are generated that can be more variable than those in isolated cells. Systems biologists Aneta Koseka and Phillipe Bastiaens have explained how, in that way, cell variety and identity are established not through genetic information, but 'in a cognitive manner'. Cells have 'individuated' through interaction with others and a higher-intelligence system has emerged.

Communication between cooperating cells is what we most think of as physiology. In more evolved species, cells become tissues to form distinct organs. Each organ is itself a multi-component system with its own structural complexity and dynamic regulations. Local communication between cells continues, but it is now nested within a wider, hierarchical system. That makes them much more sensitive to changes in the outside world, and also able to coordinate responses for the general good.

Since their emergence, multicellular creatures have evolved in a prodigious creativity of forms and lifestyles, and in an equal diversity of habitats. Relatively early were 10,000 species of sponges; 10,000 species of Cnidaria (hydra, jellyfish, sea anemones, and corals); 20,000 species of flatworms; 12,000 species of annelids (from which the common earthworm evolved); hundreds of thousands of species of molluscs; and many, many more, all coping with challenges in different corners of the world where single cells would not survive. Each new species added to the speed and variety of change in the process, stirring up a spiral of ever more complex challenges and opportunities for those that followed. It would not have been possible, or even initiated, without intelligent systems to coordinate them.

Some interesting evidence of that lies in the life history of parasites. These are the bugs, flukes, worms, and so on that live off the fruits of others' intelligent systems. Their ancestors were once as complex as the rest, but present a kind of evolution of intelligent systems in reverse. By living off their hosts' intelligent systems they no longer need all of their own. In consequence, parasites have tended to degenerate from their original to simpler forms. In some cases, multicellular forms have even reverted to a single-celled existence. So, let's take a closer look at what they've given up.

Physiology: The Intelligence of Multicellular Organisms

Cell signalling, gene transcription, and so on all become more complicated in multicellular animals. The cell does not exist independently in a changing environment, but in a changing profusion of signals from other cells, collectively dealing with the changing outside world. Physiology in single cells is through molecular networks, whereas multiple cells are embedded in wider networks *between* cells, coordinated through new layers of feed-forward/feedback loops.

One result is the absolute need, in any one cell, for signals from others. Laboratory studies have shown that without these signals all cell activity stops. It is signals *between* cells that 'tell' each cell what to do, and so coordinate the whole. The distribution of signals in space and time, and interactions between them, provide valuable information in the form of correlational patterns. From those patterns comes the intelligence for anticipation of change and predictability.

Some of that communication remains fairly local, through special junctions between neighbouring membranes. Some is more long-distance, through a variety of signalling proteins called cytokines. At one level cytokines are analogues to the inducers active in the aggregation of social bacteria and slime moulds. Later in evolution they came to operate at another level: signalling between tissues in a wider variety of functions, where they are called endocrines (or hormones). Typically, they bind to membrane receptors on target cells to induce some response beneficial to the whole system.

Physiological systems have evolved dramatically with the demands of more complex habitats. In primitive pond-dwelling multicellular organisms like *Volvox* (little more than a ball of cells with a mouth and a gut), physiology is relatively simple. With more evolved forms there is much greater differentiation into a greater number of tissues and specialised organs, and already impressive depths of coordination.

Not a Machine

In trying to understand how this coordination operates, it has been tempting to reach for mechanical metaphors. In the nineteenth century, French physiologist Claude Bernard and others suggested that physiology functions to nullify internal and external fluctuations, thus maintaining a relatively stable and benign internal milieu. Bernard's idea of 'homeostasis' was popularised by physiologist Walter Cannon in the 1930s, and is summarised in his book, *The Wisdom of the Body*. He viewed organisms as resisting environmental change and perturbation through feedback systems around set points, always returning the system to an optimum state. The upshot, he said, is that 'all of the organs in a living body act in reciprocal harmony such that separation of any individual part disturbs the entire organism'. Others, like American biologist Curt Richter, did a variety of experiments on animals to confirm the nullification of perturbations through feedback processes.

The simple, but seductive, picture of homeostasis continues to be embraced by many biologists and psychologists today. There is still a tendency to think of physiology in mechanical terms of reflexive or automatic processes with feedback loops, like your room thermostat. So it has been easy to think of physiology as merely reactive to specific fluctuations and one-off hazards, using built-in homeostatic rules and feedback systems. A kind of 'thermostat' in the hypothalamus in the brain, for example, regulates body temperature by inducing panting or shivering; dehydration creates thirst and a thirst-quenching response; animals hibernate in cold conditions and wake up in the spring, and so on – the examples are numerous.

But there are many indications that things are not so simple. One of these is that external environments rarely change as single, independent variables. For example, temperature change is usually preceded or accompanied by other changes, such as humidity or daylight levels. And that's certainly the case with internal environments, as we have seen. Such correlation patterns can foster a more anticipatory role of physiology. Accordingly, a broader view of physiology has emerged in which organisms have acquired anticipatory or pre-emptive control over changes. In a paper about brain physiology in 2020 in *Proceedings of the National Academy of Sciences (USA)*, Ryan V. Raut and associates referred to such 'adaptively regulating homeostasis' as 'allostasis'. It requires, at some level, they say, an internal predictive model of the correlation patterns in sensory inputs, including those generated from the organism's own actions. That's what I've been describing as intelligent systems.

It means that organisms don't wait for change and then react (hoping for the best). They anticipate change and pre-empt it. For example, it has been shown that there is anticipatory regulation of the heartbeat *in advance* of expected physical exertion. Animals eat if food is available to pre-empt hunger; or, in anticipation of future shortages, they fatten up. When presented with cues indicating that they are about to encounter a cold environment, animals raise their body temperature in anticipation. These suggest an intelligent system at work, now at the physiological level. This is illustrated particularly in the functioning of hormones.

Hormones Work in Concert

Long-range signalling occurs with hormones through the endocrine system. Hormones are produced by specialised tissues or glands, and their signals are mediated through hormone receptors on cell membranes. Many are associated with the brain's sensitivity to changes in the outside world and corresponding adjustments of the inside world, so they are often referred to as neuroendocrine systems. Hormones are released by the brain in response to environmental changes, triggering further hormone release by endocrine glands. The hormones circulate in the bloodstream and bind to receptors on target cells. The resulting complex is then drawn into the nucleus to adjust cell processes, including gene utilisation, as described in Chapter 3.

It is tempting to think of each of these as independent, cue–response, homeostatic systems. But they all need to be coordinated in a way sensitive to wider contexts. Hormones rarely exert effects independently in a mechanical fashion. As also described in Chapter 3, they tend to interact at the cellular level with each other and with other factors. Such contingent sensitivity can drastically alter what happens in cells and tissues. This often makes life difficult for physicians.

Coordinated Adaptability

Physiology also creates adaptability to longer-term environmental changes and conditions. It is not a set of fixed processes. The familiar examples are adaptations to extreme cold, heat, or altitude. Long-term training (or repetitive physical work) induces physiological changes that increase production of muscle fibres with enhanced blood supply. Mountaineers exploring high altitudes suffer from low oxygen levels (hypoxia). That kicks off a cell cycle that transiently increases the activity of chemoreceptors that are sensitive to oxygen levels in arteries. The result is to raise ventilation capacity and oxygen absorption in lungs and, in turn, oxygen in the arterial blood. Research has shown that high-altitude exposure of three weeks or more significantly increases lung capacity for oxygen absorption.

The neuroendocrine stress axis – or to give it it's full name, the hypothalamic–pituitary–adrenal axis (HPA axis) – is a key physiological system in adaptability. It regulates responses to stress, from internal or external sources, and also affects many body functions such as digestion, the immune system, energy metabolism, and emotional aspects of psychology (i.e. feelings). The classic stress response consists of coordinated release of a cocktail of hormones triggered by the brain through the hypothalamus. These include corticotropin, followed by cortisol, creating feelings of alarm, muscle tension, increased heart rate, and so on.

However, there are many other players in the stress–response system. One is noradrenaline (promoting a state of excitement and awareness). Another is adrenaline, released from the adrenal cortex into the bloodstream, again following stimulation by the brain. Together these produce the classic preparation for 'fight or flight', including increased heart and respiratory rates, dilation of arteries to muscles, constriction of blood flow elsewhere, release of blood sugar for energy, increase in blood pressure (to get blood to the muscles), and suppression of the immune system.

As with intelligent physiology generally, a mechanical, reflex-like 'stress–response' concept has turned out to be too simplistic. Rather than homeostasis around a fixed state, response criteria can change, depending on individual histories and current contexts. Under normal conditions that means the system managing stress in creative ways. As Marian Joëls and Tallie Baram put it in *Nature Reviews Neuroscience* in 2010, it 'results in the stress instruments producing an orchestrated "symphony" that enables fine-tuned responses to diverse challenges'. Chronic, difficult-to-manage stress, on the other hand, can have dis-harmonious psychological and neurological consequences in animals and humans. They may include emotional upset, panic attacks, post-traumatic stress disorder, and many other states. This is another aspect of human psychological performance I will return to in later chapters.

In sum, adaptability in such multi-contingent, multi-level systems occurs through assimilation of correlational patterns, as with any intelligent system. For example, cardiologist Ary Goldberger has shown how variation in the healthy human heartbeat has a deeper statistical structure, even under resting conditions. His analyses suggest that equilibrium, or maintaining constancy, is not the goal of physiological control. 'Mode locking' around a single steady state, he says, would restrict the functional adaptability of the organism. Conversely, it is the breakdown in such deeper, integrative responsiveness to changing conditions that produces disease states. Those, like narrowing of arteries and veins, high blood pressure, the ageing process, and so on, compromise the physiological dynamics. More generally, disease and aging are associated with the loss of interactions among components or component networks.

Rhythms

We all experience a more obvious example of intelligent physiology every day: that of day–night fluctuations in activity, known as circadian rhythms. All living things on earth follow day–night patterns in their behaviour. Researchers have been fascinated by them. A long time ago I camped in the lab for tiring 24-hour-plus periods to monitor aspects of the biochemistry in rat brains (and achieving my first *Nature* paper). For a long time it was thought that these continual adjustments must be part of a feedback loop driven by so-called 'clock' genes. It cannot be pinned down to a single deterministic agent, though: circadian rhythms are now known to arise spontaneously in mixtures of certain proteins and energy sources in the test tube, and they occur in red blood cells, which lack a genome altogether. Wider interactions between networks must be involved.

That is illustrated by the way the rhythms need to be regularly retuned as the day–night patterns change with the seasons, or organisms migrate (or we move to another part of the world). Now the correlation patterns among daylight, temperature, and so on, and time of day depend on a still deeper pattern (Figure 4.2). That periodic resetting of circadian rhythm affects almost every biological process in cells and organisms, including the recruitment of most genes in the genome. Seasonal changes in birdsong, for example, involve dramatic volume changes of entire brain regions in response to changing light conditions. That affects circulating levels of sex steroids and changes in behaviour. Humans blame 'seasonal affective disorder' (SAD) on diminished light and hormonal consequences in the winter months.

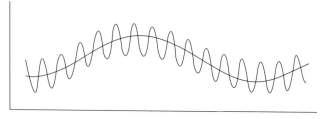

Figure 4.2 Intelligent physiology: one variable (day–night rhythms in one of many functions) conditioned by another (seasonal rhythms).

As before, these are not merely reactive but also anticipatory systems. Plants get their photosynthetic processes together, with their leaves ready-lifted, just *prior* to the onset of dawn. In animals, coordination of a whole spectrum of functions from sensitisation of chemoreceptors (as in taste and smell) and digestive systems, to tension of limb muscles, takes place just before dawn. In humans the sharpest rise in blood pressure occurs around 6.30 a.m.

In this familiar setting, 'systemic' rhythms help structure other adaptations to the deeper patterns of the seasons. But other rhythmic backgrounds have been found to scaffold intelligent processes in many aspects of life. Pulses of gene transcription (rather than steady streams) help establish patterns in development, as in the repeating segments of the earthworm, or the vertebrae of mammals. Background oscillations (high-frequency nerve pulses) in the nervous system are known to scaffold the important business of detecting and integrating correlations in the networks. Indeed, what used to be thought of as merely noise is now more positively recognised as 'stochastic resonance'.

Note, again, that there is no overall supervisor or executive officer in those dynamics. They consist of self-organising processes in a wider system of feed-forward/feedback loops. In periodically adjusting the structure of interaction between local and global networks, the whole is 'learning' new rules with wider adaptability to change. In Chapter 1 I mentioned how those IQ testers who claim to be measuring 'physiology' are mistaken. Physiology is not a quasi-mechanical system in which individual differences can be reduced to differences in 'strength' or power. Instead, we can see how a mutually compensating, dynamic system operates, and how a single 'score' of individual differences would not only be futile, but misleading. And we are still only talking about an intelligent system at an early evolutionary level.

Behaviour

Physiological intelligence facilitated the evolution of vastly more complex organisms. But more complex conditions demanded faster, even more adaptable systems. Altering anatomical and physiological states was one way. A quicker way of changing unfavourable conditions and/or finding better ones is to change location. Behaviour, and the nervous systems to control it, became that new platform for intelligence and survival.

Behaviour, in fact, probably emerged as an instrument of life-long adaptability very early in the evolution of living things. It is changes in behaviour that have, above all else, determined the course of evolution of animals over the last hundreds of millions of years. Yet poor understanding of the evolutionary status of behaviour – and especially of how it is organised – has created enduring problems.

One of those is the assumption, on the part of behavioural biologists and psychologists, that it's somehow 'in the genes'. That has meant focusing on relatively stereotyped or 'instinctive' behaviours, evolved for recurring environments: in other words, proving behaviours to be 'adaptations'. Another problem – one that pervades studies of intelligence in general – is the assumption of mechanical models. As Alex Gomez-Marin and Asif A. Ghazanfar put it in the journal *Neuron* in 2020: 'When animals are treated as passive stimulus–response, disembodied and identical machines, the life of behavior perishes.' A better understanding of intelligence helps overcome these misconceptions.

Even simple behaviour fostered survival in more rapidly changing conditions. But it started an amazing spiral in the evolution of intelligence. As animals became more mobile it made their worlds *increasingly* changeable. Even other objects appear to change by moving to, away, and around them – and increasingly so as the world filled with other behaving animals. This is a world in a different league of changeability from that of the first primitive organisms.

That's where nervous systems entered the scene. Nervous systems are, in fact, a natural evolutionary progression of physiological systems, reflecting a continuity of function. That function is the abstraction of still deeper correlation patterns in space and time.

Making sense of that new level of change required more than membrane receptors, squirms, and wriggles. Only those organisms evolving distance receptors – such as eyes and ears, faster forms of motion, and means of coordinating responses – could survive. In the maelstrom of vast numbers of variables, rapidly changing in space and time, those early pioneers of behaviour needed to be able to abstract the correlational patterns among them. So brains, too, soon evolved.

Nervous Systems

Most scientists agree that circuits of interconnected neurons probably arose around 600 million years ago. It involved specialisation of pre-existing physiological systems. Instead of 'broadcast' or loosely diffusing signals, those from some cells produced more direct outputs than others, speeding up signalling and response. Those cells that merged into networks, or nerve nets, could better coordinate signals and responses.

First came the simple nerve nets seen in animals like jellyfish, consisting of 'polymodal' neurons. They could both receive signals directly from sensory receptors on the outer surface *and* send signals to contractile ('muscle') tissues to initiate motion. Marine sponges today have such networks, and rhythmic signals along them coordinate responses. The stretchy, tentacled, pond-dwelling *Hydra*, only half a centimetre in length, clearly have nerve nets and singular sense organs (Figure 4.3). Recent research shows that stinging cells (cnidocytes) in *Hydra* tentacles, which the animals use for self-protection and to catch prey, are linked via a simple nervous system that includes primitive light-responsive cells. Together, they coordinate their feeding behaviour.

The distinctive feature of nervous systems is signalling that is fast and well-targeted. It is mediated through small chemical neurotransmitters passed across specialised terminals and onto receptors at so-called synapses. Even the simple nervous system of *Hydra* contains a repertoire of such

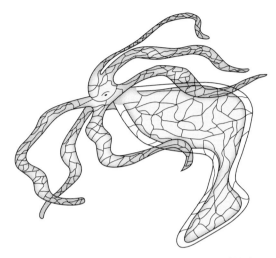

Figure 4.3   Primitive nervous system: the nerve net of *Hydra.*

neurotransmitters, as in more evolved nervous systems. New techniques, recording impulses directly from cells, have provided evidence of integration of information in *Hydra* nerve nets, over and above simple stimulus–response reflexes. It suggests abstraction of correlational intelligence even here. There is also some evidence that the networks, as a result of that, can 'rewire' or learn from experience.

By the time of the evolution of roundworms around 500 million years ago, neurons were organised in small, but definite, brains. Many examples survive today. *Caenorhabditis elegans* is a soil-dwelling nematode, similar to the potato eelworm, only 1 mm in length and with a nervous system of only 302 neurons. But it can produce highly adaptable behaviour, including associative learning and memory. For example, it can register correlations between the presence of food and environmental stimuli, such as odours, water-soluble chemicals, and temperature.

Describing what the neurons individually do, and how they 'wire up' was a stunning recent success. Even in a brain so simple, however, there is still no direct mapping of wiring to function, such as you might expect to find in a machine. Early guesses about the flow of information were largely mistaken. In other words, a precise wiring diagram does not reveal what even a tiny brain does. It is not an input/output machine detached from individual history; something more abstract is going on that a direct picture of the wiring doesn't tell us about. Even here, a 'test' describing behavioural differences could not claim to be one of 'efficiency'. So, what is the network really doing?

Network Function

We get a clue about what nervous systems do – and their connections with intelligence – from their organisation. Instead of broadcasting hormones, the signals are now channelled down long extensions (axons) to specialised connections (synapses) on shorter fibres (dendrites) of receiving cells. The signals are in the form of trains of short, sharp electro-chemical pulses, or 'action potentials', which are much faster at reaching targets (Figure 4.4).

Neurons used to be thought of as autonomous units, doing much of the decision-making for behaviour. But they form synapses on potentially hundreds or thousands of other cells, sending signals to them and receiving from just as many. We now know that dendrites are not just relay stations. More importantly, they collectively integrate the statistical (correlation) patterns arriving from the large numbers of inputs. Connections become modified in the process, enhancing or inhibiting further signals, and the neuron is assimilated into wider adaptability. It would be wrong to think of signals in nervous systems as independent stop–go signals, or as singular 'nerve impulses'. The crucial information consists of a space–time pattern of numerous impulses to and from myriad sources at once: a 'tune' rather than a single note.

Even in the brains of insects and spiders, with a few hundred to a few thousand neurons, a staggering depth of statistical structure can thus be captured for predictability and behaviour. Advanced systems have millions of cells connecting with thousands of others through billions of connections (of which, more in Chapter 6). With their enormous plasticity, changes in the world are thus continuously tracked and futures anticipated. It's not a system built for routine, mechanical computations on predictable data.

(a)

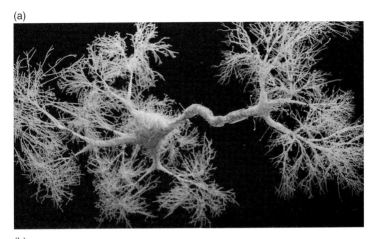

(b)

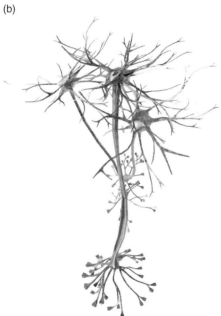

Figure 4.4 (a) A single brain cell (neuron) showing branching axon and dendrites tree; (b) a simplified illustration of how neurons form connections in networks (koto_feja/E+/ Getty Images and VICTOR HABBICK VISIONS/Science Photo Library/Getty Images).

A New Intelligence: Why?

Clearly, even the most primitive brains produce more than mechanical reflexes or routine computations. The evolution of roundworms was followed by an explosion in numbers of species. Animals started confronting and eating each other in large numbers. The major challenges for behaviour thus shifted from the physical, inanimate, world to include the *living* world. That also means change that is partly, but continually, created by animals' own activities. Survival demanded new powers for wringing predictability out of change, as in stalking, hiding, camouflaging, quick-reaction escapes, surprise attacks, and so on. Participants needed more acute perceptual and sensorimotor systems, with powers of swift discrimination and mobility. This could only be done through assimilation of more complex, statistically 'deeper' correlation patterns, dictating the conditions for the evolution of the new intelligent system in a brain.

The pattern-assimilation function evolved very early, and has been described even in the miniature brains of insects. Bees probably appeared on the planet about the same time as flowering plants, at least 90 million years ago. The brain of the honeybee has fewer than one million neurons. But it clearly abstracts complex correlation patterns. After foraging trips, bees don't find their way home by simply retracing their outward meanderings: they use the relations between landmarks, sun position, and patterns of polarised light, along with motion cues, to construct the most direct route, as if having acquired deeper statistical patterns. For example, in one study, bees were trained to forage at two feeding sites: one only in the morning at 630 metres from the hive and 115° north; the other only in the afternoon at 790 metres from the hive and 40° north. The bees were subsequently released at the 'wrong' site, either the afternoon site in the morning or vice versa. They nevertheless flew back to the hive in a direct line.

Bees visit hundreds of flowers in gathering food, inspecting potential new nest sites, learning and memorising their locations, and communicating with others through a language called the 'waggle dance'. They learn categories based on general properties such as 'vertical' and 'horizontal', still a basic cognitive function in advanced systems, as we shall see. And they must productively engage with the seething yet somehow orderly social activities in the hive.

This kind of ability suggests that bees have internalised the 'higher order' relations of the layout of the world. This kind of learning is no simple cue–response function. Biologist Miriam Lehrer, who has been studying bees for decades, says that it reflects 'a dynamic and self-organizing process of information storage'. Other research over the last few years has revealed previously unsuspected complexity of cognitive processing in invertebrates generally. In other words, the nervous system that evolved to coordinate behaviour was already fostering the emergence of a new intelligent system – a *cognitive* system.

I will have much more to say about cognitive systems in Chapter 6. But it is such a system, I suggest, that really set the pattern for the sequence that was to follow in dazzling varieties of form and function. Darwin himself famously admitted that natural selection from random variations might not be the only path to evolution. As early as 1904, Hugo De Vries was pointing out that natural selection does not explain 'the arrival of the fittest'; that natural selection is 'only a sieve . . . and not a direct cause of improvement'. Nothing can be selected until it already exists. In his book, *Arrival of the Fittest*, evolutionary biologist Andreas Wagner explains: 'Natural selection can preserve innovations, but it cannot create them. Nature's many innovations – some uncannily perfect – call for natural principles that accelerate life's ability to innovate.'

The anticipatory functions of intelligent systems fit the bill. They create variation and novel adaptations far more frequently and fruitfully than hypothetical genetic mutations could. In their emergence in nerve networks and brains they set the scene for much of what was to follow.

5   Intelligent Development

Aldous Huxley was not alone in pointing to 'the most incredible miracles happening all around us … a cell in nine months multiplies its weight thousands and thousands of times and is a child'. Indeed, development strikes everyone as a wonderful, but mysterious, transformative process in which an insignificant speck of matter becomes a coherent, functional being. It all seems so automatic as to look like magic.

That seeming mystery has been a fertile field for the imputation of hidden forces at work. Biologists and psychologists still tend to think of an immature organism 'unfolding' (a common metaphor) from a predetermined form in genes. So we may think of the development of intelligence, and of individual differences in it, as essentially 'there' already. It has also been called pre-formationism, suggesting that development is just a question of carrying out a built-in programme. Doing so may be more or less attenuated by a good or bad environment, of course. And random forces or 'noise' may play a part. But the dominant message about development remains in the usual cliches: it's genetic, innate, hard-wired, programmed, and so on.

Strangely enough, nobody has ever described a causal map, or programme, from genes to complex bodies, functions, and individual differences. It's as if deeper preconceptions compel us to think that way. It's called determinism, and adherence to it leaves us not only with poor understanding of intelligence, but also of its development. On the contrary, I have been suggesting how intelligent systems are based on pattern abstractions – that is, assimilation of complex correlations in experience. Here I show how development is itself an intelligent system in the same way, and on many different levels. I will show how the fertilised egg inherits far more than its parents' genes. It includes a whole developmental system: not a blueprint, but a construction complex facing unpredictable circumstances.

In addition, I will expand some more on connections between development and evolution. We have tended to think of development as merely an expression of past evolution, reconstructing in each generation what has been laid down by natural selection. In many ways, though, it's the other way around: development has actually come to direct evolution. The latest insights into that are described by Wallace Arthur in *Evo-Devo*. I hope to show in this chapter how development both involves and creates intelligent systems.

Why Development?

As the simple, easier ways of life became filled, living things evolved in more complex and changeable environments with more adaptable forms. Multicellularity evolved in animals, plants, and fungi as a way to survive in complex environments. Here, I focus mainly on multicellular *animals* (also known as Metazoa) in which development starts with the fusion of sperm and egg to form a zygote, the fertilised egg cell. From that, adult form and function develop.

Fertilised eggs constitute vulnerable beginnings in dicey conditions. In many respects, they don't know exactly what they are getting into until actually experienced. That's also why development is starkly different for different features and functions. As is obvious, some aspects of development, especially anatomical ones, end more or less in early adulthood. Their functions, as in vital organs, limbs, and so on, are then set up for life. At the other extreme, other aspects of development, such as learning and behaviour, are life-long and constantly changing. Those are the more complex, and more interesting, aspects. Let us start with some of the simpler details and pick up on the bigger points as we go along. I will concentrate on what happens in early development first, in a typical mammal like a human being. Some of the complications will be introduced in due course.

One Becomes Many

As we all know, animals have special organs – the ovaries and testes – for reproduction. Within the linings of those organs are produced the 'germ cells' (gametes) giving rise to eggs (ova) in females or sperm (spermatozoa) in males. In the 'somatic' cells of the body generally, the genes are arranged on chromosomes, and all cells have a full complement (i.e. pairs) of chromosomes (23 pairs for humans). In the germ cells the pairs have been separated to leave only one copy of each pair in each egg or sperm. During reproduction they are brought together at conception to form the fertilised egg, or zygote.

Then development starts, from one cell into many, with bewildering speed. A day or two after fertilisation, the egg is already rapidly dividing to form a ball of 2, 4, 8, and then 16 cells, even before implantation in the wall of the womb. Of course, this process would produce an ever-growing ball of identical cells, with identical genes, if it were not regulated in some way. It's obvious that the (identical) cells in that growing ball soon become different from one another in appropriate ways: that's the process of differentiation. Many different types of cells, each with different form and function, emerge as the beginnings of body parts. They also move to just the right places at just the right times, in an orchestrated manner. That presents the puzzle of how genetically identical cells can 'know' how to become one of so many different kinds, and where to move to.

Quite distinctly, as seen under a microscope, the ball of cells hollows out to become a fluid-filled sac, called the blastocoel. The cells now surrounding it – collectively called the blastula – have the amazing capacity to become any cell type and tissue in the adult body. These are the pluripotent stem cells. They soon change into cells of different sizes, shapes, and types to form three new layers – the ectoderm, mesoderm, and endoderm – of the gastrula. Figure 5.1 illustrates the process in simplified form in the sea urchin embryo.

A bewildering variety of cells types and tissues arises from these layers. Figure 5.2 shows just a few of them. Those from one small area of the gastrula – called the neural tube – creep in different directions to become diverse neurons of the brain; sensory neurons of touch, smell, hearing, and

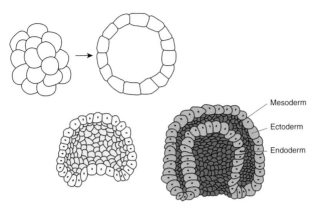

Figure 5.1 Early cell division and formation of gastrula with three differentiated layers.

vision; endocrine cells (producing hormones); various cardiac tissue cells; pigment cells of the skin; and internal organs and blood vessels. Cells from the neural tube also give rise to facial bone and cartilage, the cornea of the eye, meninges (membranes around the brain), roots for teeth and eye muscles, and many others. And this is all from one originally tiny clump of cells in a tiny area of the gastrula.

This is creation of numbers and varieties of cells on a colossal scale. Over the period of a few weeks over 30 *trillion* (yes, trillion) cells of 200 different kinds are produced. If they were footballs they would swamp the earth. But that's not all: it also involves massive migrations over long distances so that they end up in the right place at just the right time to form the different tissues. That's the equivalent of thousands of miles in human terms.

Every cell in the body, from the backbone and gut to the brain, and from the tips of the fingers to the tips of the toes, has arisen from this swarming of multitudes from a common starting place. And it's happened with astonishing order and harmony and predictability. It's little wonder there is talk of miracles, or that such a highly integrated and harmonious process must be under the close supervision of some very clever designer that already 'knows' what to do in great detail. The genes and genetic programmes

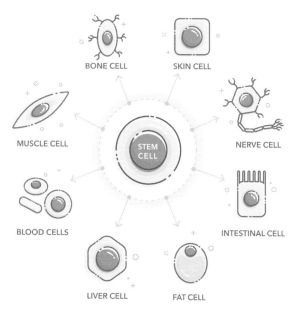

Figure 5.2   Stem cells develop and differentiate into many different types (DrAfter123/DigitalVision Vectors/Getty Images).

are the usual suspects. Yet all those cells have the same genes. And those are merely sequences of nucleotides, blind as to outcomes. They cannot be the prime movers; they are merely accessories (in fact convenient molecular templates). So let's see where the intelligence for this miracle really comes from.

Knowing What to Become

The process is analogous with what happened when single cells evolved into multicellular creatures, though on a vastly more complex scale (see Chapter 4). In development, as in evolution, differentiation of cells is based on 'outside' structure taken 'inside'. As a single cell, the young egg may look like a homogeneous sphere. But the apparent uniformity is already rendered uneven, or structured, by several factors. For example, the point of entry of the sperm cell provides the egg with polarity – an anterior and posterior (or a front and a rear). The point of attachment to the wall of the womb may be another.

More importantly, the mother has deposited a host of messages of her own in the egg. These include products of her own genes: transcription factors, which recruit genes; promoters, which tell them when to start transcription; enhancers, which regulate how much; and a rich cellular milieu of RNAs, proteins, fats, sugars, vitamins, metal salts, and so on. In addition, the mother has placed chemical 'locks' on some of her offspring's genes, influencing, from her own experience, how those genes should be used. This is part of what is known as 'epigenetics' – a way in which some parental experiences, as well as their genes, are passed on to the child. Finally, the sperm has deposited its own cargo of active ingredients at a specific location.

All of these ingredients are unevenly distributed. In consequence, when the egg divides, some of the daughter cells will contain more of some of those biochemical constituents than others. Those different concentrations are information for the cells about what to do in response to other signals from outside.

Morphogen Harmonies

Also, right from the start, the stem cells are raining storms of signals on each other. These are every bit as numerous and detailed as the radio signals that saturate the airwaves in our modern communications, only here they are chemical messages reaching surface receptors on other cells. Hitting a receptor results in signal registration. A further signal is then passed to the inside of the cell, and activation of metabolic responses follows. Of course, a thousand cells shooting out such signals to others, crowded into a small space, all at the same time, sounds more like bedlam than intelligent development. But it's not isolated signals that a cell is listening out for, any more than a bird is listening for a specific note in the dawn chorus or a bat detects a single frequency in its echo-location system. Rather, it's the shape of the space–time patterns within the storm that turns it all from cacophony to harmony.

Revealing what that chemical chatter and the patterns within it consist of has been a slow, but exciting, process. In a famous paper in 1952, the wartime code-breaker Alan Turing suggested that it's the *concentration gradients* of the signals that constitute the important information. The idea is that the signals secreted by cells diffuse through the tissues of the embryo. The concentration of each signal diminishes with distance from the point of release. Every other cell is thus given some positional information in relation to the transmitter, according to place in the gradient. Cells close to the source will receive the signal in higher concentrations and respond one way. Those further away will receive it in low concentrations and respond in another way. Such chemical 'morphogens' were in fact soon discovered, and the theory was elaborated by Lewis Wolpert and Francis Crick in the 1960s and 1970s.

The whole process is incredibly intricate, however. Obviously, there are multiple gradients from multiple morphogens being secreted simultaneously. That creates cross-cutting gradients, themselves dynamically patterning in space and time: a three-dimensional moving tapestry, if that can be imagined. Interactions between the gradients, their timing, duration, and where they reach cell surfaces all influence what goes on within each cell, including what genes to utilise and when. Nor is the traffic one-way. It's now known that a pool of undifferentiated stem cells maintain feed-forward signals to those differentiating, while the latter keep on signalling to each other *and* feeding back signals to their parent pool. These are further examples of classic feed-forward/feedback loops in intelligent systems, here steering the ongoing fates of cells in a new level of developmental intelligence.

Finally, other 'guidance factors' have been discovered, secreted from some cells to 'pull' others towards them in widescale migrations. These are particularly important in arrangements of neurons and the growth of nerve fibres (axons) onto their correct targets. It can all seem like the fading in and out of the different instruments in an orchestra, with their precise intersection in time and harmonious consequences. But there is no conductor and no written music. The patterning of development emerges with great precision, while conferring robustness against many bumps and hazards. Biologist Brian Goodwin spoke of a 'self-organised entity' born out of the 'relational order' between myriad players on this very complex stage. Development is 'dancing to the tune of life', as Denis Noble puts it.

Those emergent tunes or dances – more than the sums of their parts – are the intelligence of development. Over a matter of hours and days the first cells have started to differentiate into hundreds of different kinds. The essential body structures – body axis and segments, brain, limbs, and organs – soon begin to form under the dynamics of local interactions. But the course of development is not the same for all features and functions. Some, like limbs, organs, or overall body plan, seem to follow a relatively uniform course. Others, like muscle bulk, aspects of physiology, and, as we now know, brain networks, are far more modifiable. Correspondingly, it was noticed long ago that large environmental changes seem to have little effect on some traits, while small changes can have enormous (if not always immediate) effects on others. The developmental intelligence seems to 'think' differently for different characteristics. But that all makes sense in the context of environmental change.

Sticking to a Course

In experiments in the 1940s, in Edinburgh, developmental biologist Conrad Waddington discovered that the development of many characteristics strongly resists deviation from a specific course. Developing embryos experience many bumps and shocks, and have variable genes, that, theoretically, could cause such deviations. Yet there are many examples of fairly standard, workable, forms and functions developing in all individuals, regardless. Waddington used the term 'canalisation' to describe the process. He realised it must be due to factors other than rigid genetic programmes, and coined the term 'epigenetics'.

Such robustness makes sense. The characteristics so buffered tend to be those crucial for survival in circumstances that typically recur across generations. They include physical characteristics such as eyes and limbs, key organs, and physiological processes. Offspring will need them just like their parents did, so sticking to the course is vital. Canalisation has to do with meeting demands that recur across generations, in spite of immediate bumps and shocks.

If that mountain-top radio mast simply must be erected where gales, blizzards, or avalanches are all possible, make sure your plans are resilient enough to stay the course. You will need sensitive feed-forward/feedback loops in measurements, organisation, and inter-worker communications. That's the intelligence of canalised traits.

Canalisation is also evident at the behavioural level. It includes a variety of simple reflexes, and all the stereotyped mating, nesting, defensive, migration, and other patterns of behaviour that we often call 'instincts'. Like the casual observer, many biologists and psychologists easily think of such forms, functions, and behaviours as 'innate': surely, the scheming of genetic programmes? But that's not the case: all are as much the fruits of developmental intelligence as is the prodigious flowering of cellular variation described above.

Sets of co-evolved molecular components have been discovered that foster that more 'closed' development, even in behaviour patterns. Through their interactions those components can continually correct deviations and maintain direction. The interactions will recruit specific genes as and when needed. But those genes are used as resources for the development of behaviours, not as designers, so development of the correct numbers of legs and arms, 32 teeth, 2 eyes and ears, and so on, will be the same across generations. And the intelligent result is few, if any, important individual differences.

Just how interactive and mutually compensatory such networks are has been well demonstrated in the laboratory, using various chemical tools. In experiments in fruit flies, for example, it has been necessary to disrupt many pathways at once to produce any variation in development. When disruption *is* achieved – that is, the compensatory interactions are disrupted – spectacular things happen. Huge, and often monstrous, differences in anatomies and physiologies, previously showing little or no variation, suddenly appear. (Your radio mast goes up – but as tangled structures of metal and wire.) This indicates how robust the evolved networks are under wide variations of genes and environments.

Choosing Alternatives

Not all characteristics and their development are like that because many aspects of environments change across generations. In the simplest cases that may mean a change in single factors like temperature, available nutrients, presence of predators, and so on, which were not experienced by parents. Then, canalised development could produce misfits. Instead, development needs to be more adaptable, or *plastic*. That means delaying development until the actual environment has been encountered.

Developmental plasticity has been exhaustively studied in simple animals. A popular illustration is that of the water flea, *Daphnia*. If juveniles develop in the same pool of water as a predatory midge larvae (*Chaoborus*), they develop a protective 'neck spine' or 'helmet'. These defensive structures allow the *Daphnia* to escape from their predators more effectively. However, they are completely absent in parents (or other offspring) that developed in predator-free water. The developmental network has evolved sensitivity to some chemical hormones (kairomones) inadvertently released by the predator. In its presence, the network intelligently switches development onto another track.

There are numerous examples of such plasticities, sometimes referred to as 'polyphenisms' (many forms). Wing patterns in some pupating butterflies develop according to the seasons: light if they pupate in the spring, but darker in the autumn. Jean Piaget was struck by the way water snails developing in pond habitats have elongated shells, whereas the same species developing in more turbulent lake conditions have more compact shells.

Sometimes developmental plasticity is spectacular. In the castes in bees and ants it radically alters behaviour and physiology, as well as anatomy. Locusts likewise develop distinct 'morphs' in response to current population densities. Even sex determination in some reptiles is known to be developmentally plastic. Investigators incubating alligator eggs in the laboratory were initially astonished to find that offspring were either all male or all female. It was subsequently realised that sex development was influenced by local temperature.

In many cases, developmental plasticity is time- or stage-dependent, as in the classic metamorphosis of frogs and other amphibians. Over time, we see the remodelling of almost every organ in the body, and radical changes in behaviour from filter feeder to predator, as well as form of locomotion. All that is wrought despite the same sets of genes.

Developing Brains

Of course, the most celebrated example of developmental plasticity is that in the brain. Canalised development seems to ensure that neurons in different layers in the cerebral cortex – the most recently evolved aspect of the brain – form the requisite variety of processing types and their organisation into distinct layers. These will then be 'good enough' for the demanding tasks ahead. But further organisation of brain networks into specialised areas, with their specific response properties, follows. That depends upon patterns of inputs in actual experience.

This has been demonstrated spectacularly in laboratory studies. Many years ago, neuroscientist Mriganka Sur and his colleagues did experiments on newborn ferrets. They surgically re-routed visual nerve connections from the eye away from their usual destination in the visual cortex of the brain. The nerves were directed, instead, to what usually develops as the *auditory* cortex (i.e. for hearing). That auditory cortex subsequently came to process visual information like an ordinary visual cortex. Writing in 2020 on his lab website, Mriganka Sur says that 'cortical plasticity is implemented by learning rules'; patterns of correlations assimilated from experience 'wire' the networks accordingly.

In other experiments, plugs of cortex were transplanted from, say, visual to somatosensory areas (responding to sensations of touch). The plugs developed connections characteristic of their new location, rather than of their origins. So 'visual' tissue came to process data from skin and muscles rather than eyes. Likewise, if undifferentiated embryonic neurons are transplanted to the visual cortex of adult mice, they soon take on all the anatomy and physiology of neurons typical of that area. Finally, it has been shown how the functions of one area of the brain, surgically removed, can be taken over by another.

Developmental plasticity obviously reflects variation being created by intelligent systems, rather than programmes from blind code in genes. It will be favoured when the environment is quite changeable in space and time – when predetermined programmes, or canalisation of development, would create misfits. Moreover, its 'language' – of *patterns* rather than elements – of experience, affords great economy of processing. Human and animal studies show that brain networks undergo massive synaptic 'pruning' during childhood. About half of the synapses rapidly proliferated in the womb get slowly removed, right up until puberty. This reflects the ongoing compression of specific learnings into increasingly abstract (and more adaptable) processing rules.

Life-Long Development

As we know, important environmental changes, presenting many challenges, occur throughout life for all complex organisms. One-shot developmental plasticities, with lasting effects, cannot cope with such continuous change. What is logically required for survival in such conditions are living structures and functions that can adapt to changes *throughout the life of the individual*.

All living things have evolved such functions. Indeed, they were probably there at the origins of life, as the first intelligent systems. There are many simple and familiar examples: the colour changes of the chameleon; growing protective skin calluses at points of friction; increasing muscle bulk and strength with exercise; and, in animals, changing hair/fur colour and thickening with the seasons. Some are visibly spectacular. As mentioned previously, seasonal changes in birds' brains dramatically alter song and other behaviours. Some fish can undergo a total sex reversal in which a female develops the colouration, behaviour, and gonadal physiology and anatomy of a fully functioning male. An example we tend to take for granted is that of the immune system. The system works through the kinds of signalling networks described in Chapter 3, whereby mutation rates in DNA become vastly enhanced. Entirely novel antibodies may be produced throughout the life of an individual as new bugs and toxins are encountered. Individual profiles of antibodies continually develop and vary according to life history. There is no 'best' profile.

What's happened is that developmental plasticity, normally terminating in juveniles, has been further relaxed. A higher level of intelligence emerges in the course of actual experience, throughout life. Of course, it is difficult for gross anatomical traits to switch form all the time to track changes. Instead, behaviour, learning, brains, and cognition have become more important.

I will be looking at these aspects in the next and subsequent chapters. In this chapter so far I have been trying to illustrate how development involves active intelligent systems – self-organised processes with emergent properties. Development is not the confluence of blind genomes and fortuitous (or otherwise) environments. Let us now consider some of the implications for broader views of development.

Developmental Maps?

It will always be tempting to attribute the construction of complex form to some prior programme, however invisible or elusive. Even today, some behaviour geneticists continue to look for 'maps' from genes to brains to intelligence in humans. But research over the last few decades has completely turned that idea on its head. Genetic involvement in development is *downstream* from intelligent processes, not upstream. Moreover, the products of those genes are themselves altered and used in different ways, according to developmental and metabolic needs.

Of course, even the most ardent gene hunters admit a role for environmental factors in development. But the intelligence in developmental systems isn't remotely captured in common descriptions like 'a mixture of genes and environment' or 'nature and nurture'. That's like saying a cake is a mixture of ingredients and an oven, without any role for a cook. Instead, developmentalists speak of a constructive dialogue between internal systems and the dynamics of the environment.

That's why, in fact, there is little direct mapping between differences in genes (the DNA sequences) and differences in developmental endpoints (or phenotypes). With complex traits, operating through intelligent systems, the identification of specific 'difference-makers' is problematic, except in unusual conditions (see below). As with choosing which font you type with, most genetic and associated protein variations are, except in rare circumstances, adequate. Most will do the job. Through epigenetic functions, unfortunate environmental conditions can be nullified.

The genes *do* serve as DNA templates to form the RNAs that form the proteins. But their variation or even absence is not deterministic. We saw in Chapter 3, for example, that we can get a multitude of different proteins from the same genes. Andreas Wagner and Jeremiah Wright have studied different signal-ling pathways and large metabolic networks requiring gene products. They found that the same metabolic ends could be met in various ways in spite of genetic variation. They concluded that multiple alternative pathways are the rule rather than the exception in living things. Similarly, Frederik Nijhout and colleagues analysed the genes necessary in humans for the production of the enzymes in critical metabolic pathways. They were surprised to discover that there is considerable variation in such genes. But, as they also discovered, epigenetic processes greatly reduce the effects of that variation in the functioning system.

The opposite is also true: individuals with identical sets of genes can be markedly different from one another. Embryonic stem cells, with the same genomes, develop a vast variety of identities. Likewise, a population of animals of identical genotypes, reared in identical environments, can show the full, normal range of individual differences in form and behaviour as if developing in the wild. Most laboratory animals, for example, have been bred to be genetically identical and raised in the same cage. Yet they show immense variations in physiology and behaviour, and even immune responses. This is usually put down, rather intuitively, to 'noise'. But they are likely due to the more constructive dynamics of interactions between individuals operating at many levels.

That is suggested in a famous 700-year-old herd of ancient wild cattle, or Aurochs, in Northumberland in the UK (known as the Chillingham Herd). They have become so inbred over countless generations as to be virtually genetically identical. Yet they still develop the normal range of individual differences of anatomical and behavioural characteristics. They form normal variation in social relations, joust for dominance hierarchies, have characteristic calls, and so on, just like their wild (and genetically variable) relatives.

In the brain, too, genes are needed for resources, but not as architects. Biologist Julia Freund and colleagues observed the development of genetic-ally identical mice living in one large, enriched environment. Despite the genetic and environmental uniformity, the researchers observed the emer-gence of notable individual differences in behaviour over time. These differ-ences reflected individual differences in brain structure. Again, it seemed that individuality could be attributed to factors emerging from interactions with others in the course of development.

Finally, I hinted earlier at what are now also called 'trans-generational epigenetic' effects. Through intelligent systems, environments experienced by parents can alter aspects of the genome to influence development in the next generation. This consists of leaving a molecular tag on genes that act as 'do not use' labels. The tags are inherited with the genes in the usual way. In studies of individual differences, using the simple models described in Chapter 2, variation will be mistaken as 'genetic', but it is 'non-genetic' inheritance.

In sum, trying to predict form and individual differences from a read-out of DNA, or enumeration of genes, is almost always pointless (except for the rare cases I discuss below). That is why we need to be careful in the way we speak about genetic 'causes' of development. The idea conceals a semantic minefield.

Innate or Developed?

Intelligence and instinct have traditionally been viewed as opposites: the latter created through a genetic programme; the former at least partially developed through experience, or learned (with individual differences described as 'learning ability'). But, as mentioned above, there is still confusion about the relationship between them. The difficulty dissolves, however, once we appreciate the significance of environmental context, especially its changeability.

First, there are no genetic programmes in the superstitious sense of hidden messages in genes, passed intact across generations. I hope to have now convinced readers of that. Second, so-called innate traits depend on developmental processes just as much as more plastic characteristics. What are perceived as innate are stereotyped, highly predictable, response tendencies. Often, they are triggered by specific signals from the environment: a jabbing finger invokes an eye-blink; lengthening days bring on nest-building; and so on. They appear as predetermined because they evolved to 'fit' conditions that reliably recur across generations. But they are enshrined in molecular networks in cells, inherited as constraints on development, as described for canalisation above.

As such inherited bundles, the development of even innate traits can be changed by novel or unaccustomed experience. As neuroscientist Mark Blumberg explained regarding survival instincts, migratory instincts, herding instincts, and so on, a closer look reveals that these and other instincts are not inborn, pre-programmed, hard-wired, or genetically determined: 'Rather, research in this area teaches us that species-typical behaviors *develop* – and they do so in every individual under the guidance of species-typical experiences occurring within reliable ecological contexts.' There are no mysterious designers and their programmes.

Genetic Causes

Some of this may seem strange to those with a modicum of knowledge about the history of genetics. Many of us were taught, or have read, how Gregor Mendel supposedly demonstrated associations between gene variations and trait differences in his sweet peas? Are not these 'difference-makers', and, indeed, part of the important laws of genetics? By the same token, it's surely easy to see that parents 'pass on' many of their physical characteristics: hair and eye colour, height, facial features, and so on – things that 'run in the family'. Is that not genes directing development and causing differences (and determining intelligence as much as these more obvious differences)?

Moreover, we all know of diseases statistically associated with mutations to genes, some affecting systems at various levels, including the cognitive level. These surely reflect inherited codes for development and individual differences in it? Some, such as phenylketonuria (PKU), have been known for decades, including many with substantial impacts, such as Huntington's disease and cystic fibrosis. By the start of this century, thousands of seemingly inherited diseases, attributable to rogue variants in single genes, had been described. It seems quite legitimate, in such cases, to speak of genetic causes.

Taking this last issue first: it was the big hope of gene sequencing, as in the Human Genome Project, that, by identifying such genetic causes, cures would soon be on the way. That could involve simple lifestyle changes, such as avoiding a component of diet (as with avoiding the amino acid phenylalanine in PKU). Or perhaps new drugs could help correct a deviant pathway and keep development on track. More recently, direct genetic engineering or editing has been explored: biochemically cutting out the defective variant and replacing it with a normal one.

Many statistical associations between genetic variations and specific disorders have been reported. However, establishing the causal role of those variants has not generally been straightforward. Effects tend to be weak or unpredictable. Often, many additional genes are involved and there are environmental effects. A mutation lethal in some individuals may be harmless in others. Some people with Huntington disease variants get their first symptoms at age 80, others at age 2, and most between ages 30 and 50. The same gene variants can affect different people, even in the same family, in very different ways.

All that reflects intelligent systems compensating for the resource deficiency as much as possible. As always, correlations can be predictive in a statistical sense, but do not usually provide causal understanding. And that will not come from treating the organism as a black box. In traditional experimental methods we may establish causation between two factors X and Y when it is shown that intervention on X changes the value of Y *under a range of background conditions*. That is impossible where causes are embedded in multi-level networks of interactions. Any links reported will tend to be very fuzzy.

Obviously, where development *is* being disrupted by the absence of a genetic resource, then we may suspect a 'genetic cause' or a 'genetic susceptibility' as clear difference-makers – just as we may speak of iron deficiency in the diet as a cause of anaemia. But we must recognise that this is a very specific use of the term 'cause'. We should not slip into using it as an analogy of the role of genes in creating normal form and individual differences. A loose wheel nut may vary the form and direction of travel of your car, but we should not take that as a model of causes in general. As Denis Noble has proposed, it is best to think of these as causes in a purely passive sense, with little if any implication for understanding the causes of development in general.

The same reasoning applies to the single-gene effects studied by Mendel. For example, some of his pea plants had purple flowers, while others had white.

Patterns of inheritance seemed to reflect differences in a single 'hereditary unit' (what were later called genes). So it's easy to think of a gene for white flowers and a gene (in fact a different version of the same gene) for purple flowers. Surely a genetic difference-maker?

Well, yes, so long as we remember its specific context. In fact, the statistical association obscures several streams of chemical synthesis of the purple pigment (anthocyanin), involving the products of many other genes. A tiny alteration, or mutation, in one gene (a transcription factor) disrupts this orchestration. In its *absence* the flower is white. That, too, is an illustration of 'passive causation'.

That bears also on a point mentioned in Chapter 3. Traits associated with large amounts of genetic variation are unlikely to be functionally important. With important traits, variation has either been weeded out by natural selection, or nullified by intelligent systems (such as canalisation or developmental plasticity). The traits studied by Mendel are, indeed, of little import to survival. White flowers survive as well as purple flowers. Either is good enough. Otherwise, one or the other would have been eliminated by natural selection. In consequence, we need to be careful about how we infer causes from genes, especially as 'difference-makers'. I will be discussing environment and intelligence in a wider context in Chapter 8.

Development and Evolution

In this chapter I've been trying to show how development is itself a form of intelligent system. The intelligence, as in other systems, emerges from interactions among many components guided by correlation patterns in experience. As such, development has deeper implications for how we view the evolution of living things.

The agricultural model assumes simple maps from genetic differences to differences in 'fitness' followed by natural selection. But does it explain the profusion of forms and functions we have seen in the course of evolution? There has been much debate about that. As mentioned in Chapter 4, natural selection can increase the frequency of innovations, but it cannot create them. Moreover, most complex traits – even physical ones like eyes, beaks, jaws, or limbs – are composites of many parts. Random alteration of any one part will be of no advantage. What is needed is an understanding of life's propensity to innovate.

We now know how intelligent systems may provide the basis of such understanding. They can anticipate probable futures and actively develop adaptive forms and functions. By such means, intelligent development has helped direct evolution rather than be directed by it. As Mary Jane West-Eberhard explained, development processes ensure that 'genes are followers, not leaders, in adaptive evolution'. We will see that spectacularly when we turn to human intelligence in Chapter 7.

6 Intelligent Machine?

Nearly everyone thinks that it's your brain, and how it varies from the brains of others, that defines your intelligence as an individual. The terms 'brainy' and 'intelligent' are used almost interchangeably. If you really want to know about intelligence then you need to know about the brain. You may come across questions like 'How does the brain give rise to intelligence?' or 'Where does intelligence reside in the brain?'. It is generally believed that knowing more about the brain will tell us more about intelligence, and much else, including human nature itself.

That's the main reason the brain has been under siege by researchers over the last few decades. Psychologists, educators, and even sociologists and economists, as well as neuroscientists, are all in on it. So we have the current fashion for adding the prefix *neuro-* to studies, courses, departments, and professorial titles, wherever possible. It looks and sounds as if we're really going to get intelligence pinned down. Much of the trend has aimed to paint causal pictures from gene codes to brain 'wiring' to intelligence. 'How does the genome encode behaviour through the development of the nervous system?' asked the *Royal Society* in the introduction to a talk on 16 January 2020. We are also surrounded by what's been called *neurogenetic reductionism*, or the belief that complex functions can be understood by describing their simpler components.

The trend reflects the firm belief that knowing the gene-wired brain in that way will reveal what it really is to be human. It never fails to create frissons of exciting discovery. Indeed, there has been an outpouring of sometimes dazzling, and always fascinating, findings about aspects of the brain from the thousands of neuroscience laboratories that now exist. Popularisers like Kevin Mitchell never fail to remind us that it's an 'exciting time' to be in the area; or that we are 'beginning to understand how instinct and innate preferences and behaviors are wired into the circuitry of the brain'. Others have suggested that cognitive intelligence can, in theory, be completely explained in the language and data of neurophysiology – it's just a question of time.

Many of these projects need to be cheered on, of course. But, as for 'higher' cognitive functions, the reality is a little more sobering. The truth is, there is still little consensus about how intelligence is related to the brain, except in very general terms. That's not least because of shallow or vague views about what intelligence is. We have mountains of fascinating details, but they have not yet been woven into an integrated view of what brains – from flies to humans – are really for. Well into the twenty-first century, how the brain is linked to intelligence remains a profound mystery.

One sure sign of that – as with the concept of the gene – is resort to simplistic metaphors. That's how the brain tends to be put to a naive public by brain scientists. In his book *The Idea of the Brain*, Matthew Cobb describes how we have tried to understand the brain in terms of the technologies of the period: clocks, telephones, computers, machines, and so on. The 'computational' metaphor, drawn from the digital processor, currently dominates cognitive models of intelligence. A conference on *Global Challenges for the Brain Sciences* in 2016 declared that 'Brains remain the most computationally advanced machines for a large array of cognitive tasks.' And, in his book *Intelligence and Human Progress*, James Flynn talked about 'genetic potential for a better-engineered brain', likening it to a 'high-performance sports car'.

Psychologists – especially those looking for the genes for IQ – have readily taken up the mechanical metaphors. Individual differences are reduced to differences in brain power, capacity, speed of processing, and so on (i.e. the elusive g). The result is that the brain has been pulled apart like a machine. Its components are analysed for functional clues. Centres of specialised processing are allegedly identified, as if, in order to understand intelligence, we need to understand what each part of it 'does'.

As Cobb explains, such mechanical reductions are all inadequate, and we need radical new ideas. The *Global Challenges* conference just mentioned recognised that 'understanding the design principles ... hold the key to understanding intelligence'. But its posting still admits that the subject 'remains mysterious'. For all the excitement and hype, it remains a huge problem because the properties of intelligence are emergent from interactive factors, on many levels, not those of specific components.

What the Brain Is For

To understand the scale of the problem, and for simplicity, let us concentrate on the task of dealing intelligently with a single object through the most acute of our senses, vision (though much of what I have to say will apply to other senses, too, as we shall see). Superficially, it doesn't seem too difficult to get an object image from the environment through the eye to the brain. The camera has been a potent metaphor for the process. You look at an object and can easily imagine that it can be decomposed into a set of 'features': lines, corners, angles, pixels, or whatever, just permutated in a specific way. It's also easy to suppose that the light-sensitive part of the eye – the retina – just 'picks up' those features in direct topographical form and passes them on to the brain (this is *sensory reception*). The brain then puts the pieces back together, according to some genetically wired rules or computations (this is *perception*). Other built-in operations can then be performed, like recognising, classifying, thinking, memorising, constructing motor responses, and so on (this is *cognition*).

It sounds simple. For most of us, most of the time, the process works so brilliantly that we hardly ever stop to question it. It has been a very influential view of how the brain, and our intelligence, deals with the visual world – and other sensory inputs as well. But things *aren't* so simple. Despite big efforts, says Mathew Cobb, 'we still only dimly understand what is going on when we see'.

There are many reasons why feature detection and camera-image reproduction cannot create even immediate perceptions. The first of these is that a three-dimensional object is collapsed as a two-dimensional image on the retina. Like shadows cast on a wall, the same two-dimensional image can be created by a number of different objects/features. How do we distinguish one from another? The back of the eye is also cup-shaped, so the image will be distorted. And, like the camera image, it's upside-down. More crucially, a photo or picture is a 'still', whereas the real world outside is a 'movie' – a constant flux of objects through which we, and our sensory receptors, are 'swimming' in constant motion.

In fact, the visual environment is never static. An object is commonly viewed from different angles and at different distances, under constant transformation of appearance. As it moves – or you move – to different places and distances (with changes in apparent size), the image may also rotate, pass behind other objects, be deformed (in the case of non-rigid objects), and so on. There will probably be numerous objects in the same scene, but somehow they are still identified. The brain must also distinguish that motion from the motion of the image on the retina due to eye and head movements. In the early 1900s, psychologist William James famously referred to the 'blooming, buzzing confusion' of the sensory input experienced by the infant. In the 1960s, perception psychologist James Gibson described such 'invariance under transformation' as one of the most fundamental problems in psychology.

What we do know is that we somehow get over such problems. Experimental psychologist Irving Rock called it perceptual 'problem-solving' or 'intelligent perception': that is, going beyond the information given. We have seen how simpler intelligent systems achieve just that through the abstraction of correlational patterns. That may be the real function of brains as well.

The Intelligent Solution

There is abundant evidence that (a) the visual world, like the world in general, is full of such statistical (correlation) patterns, and (b) the function of the brain, from the external senses 'inwards', is to abstract them. Clues as to how they do that come from the importance of motion in perception.

Indeed, all aspects of the world as experienced abound in the time and motion patterns that furnish predictability. Objects visually present three-dimensional structures changing in time, and therefore there are four dimensions. That vastly enhances the correlation structure. It has been shown many times that objects in motion can be recognised better and faster than static objects. Researchers of face perception have discovered how much quicker people are at recognising moving faces than static pictures. When we move around a book on a table, something invariant about its 'bookness' persists in spite of radical changes in appearance. You continue to recognise it as a book. So crucial is such *dynamic* structure that without it the world cannot be 'sensed'. If a dead fly on a string is dangled motionlessly in front of a starving frog, the frog cannot sense this meal to save its life. In humans it has been shown that the image of an object held perfectly still on the eyeball (by using a kind of contact lens) quickly fades and 'disappears'.

The importance of motion for three-dimensional shape perception was demonstrated 50 years ago by experimental psychologist Hans Wallach. In a classic experiment, participants were shown shadows of a wireframe figure as projected onto a translucent screen. They were asked to report their perceptions. They said that the image appeared flat when the wireframe is stationary, but 'pops out' in three-dimensional depth as soon as it is rotated. This is called the 'kinetic depth effect', but that only describes the effect, not how it comes about.

Not surprisingly, then, it has been shown that although the retina may *receive* points of light, what it's really interested in is the correlations between them. Indeed, the cellular organisation of the retina is that of typical feed-forward /feedback loops for doing just that. The feed-forward links are obvious. But between and across the cell layers there are also reciprocal, feedback loops in the circuitry. It means that neurons can interact laterally within the same layer, and vertically from one layer to the other (Figure 6.1).

I explained earlier what those feed-forward/feedback loops are for, and will do again later in the context of higher brain functions. That here in the retina they are already condensing data into correlational patterns is suggested in one rather stark feature: the retina contains more than 100 million photoreceptors, but there are only one million ganglion cells actually sending messages to the brain. It turns out, in other words, that what your eye 'sees', and what it tells your brain, is not like sequences of camera shots. Rather, the light elements – or 'pixels' – have been re-coded in terms of relations between them.

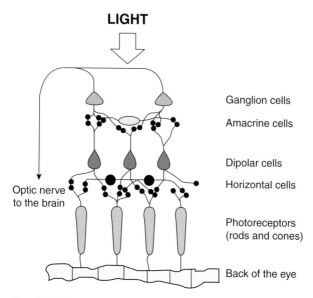

Figure 6.1   Schematic diagram of the retina and cell connections. Light strikes the back of the eye first, against which the retina is actually inverted.

By using that structure, the brain can go beyond the information given. The point is, the world is simply teeming with such correlational structure, usually including much deeper levels of nestedness or dependency. It's all fodder to an intelligent system for constructing visual intelligence in the brain. A row of two or more lights switched on in swift succession – popular in fairgrounds and theatre fronts – creates an illusion of a single light in motion. It is actually registered as true motion in certain motion-sensitive cells in the visual cortex. Similarly, two lights moving in typical space–time correlation down a highway are quickly constructed in the 'mind's eye' as a vehicle moving towards you.

One of the best illustrations is the 'point light walker', a stick-like figure of a person, in the dark, with only around a dozen lights at a few critical places

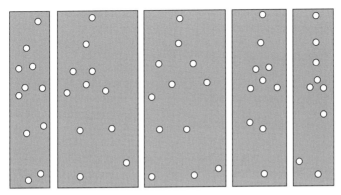

Figure 6.2 A sequence of stills from a 'point light walker'. Presentation as a sequence at normal speed evokes almost immediate recognition of a person walking.

like elbows, knees, and head (Figure 6.2). Volunteers are presented with the images against a dark background, such as on a computer screen. Individual images are not quickly recognised in static forms, but presentation as a sequence at normal speed evokes almost immediate recognition of a person walking.

In experiments on animals, recording from neurons in the brain while exposed to naturalistic stimuli (such as in videos) has also shown the dependence of recognition on higher-order correlations. Similar principles seem to apply to other sense modes. For example, it is known that receptors in the cochlea of the ear transform typical sounds into their correlational structure before sending them along the auditory nerve to the brain. Tactile senses, too, are able to abstract the deeper statistical structure from sequences of vibration across the skin.

Brain functions are based on that kind of statistical structure, and constructive inference. The brain is sometimes described as 'data hungry', whereas it is really 'pattern hungry' because it is 'predictability hungry'. By having assimilated such patterns in the networks of the brain, great predictability becomes possible. From molecular networks to brains, there is no route to predictability and intelligent activity other than by capturing relational structure. This is a better way of thinking about brain function than as the mechanical routines of a cerebral engine. It is reflected in brain structure itself.

Brain Structure

Batteries of impulses shaped in space and time are sent from the retina (and other sensory receptors) along axons to way-stations in the midbrain for further processing. Then they are sent to the cerebral cortex, the huge mantle over the rest of the brain that has expanded so prominently in the course of evolution. But the signals are not forwarded as independent spikes representing isolated features. Rather, they are sent as 'clouds' of pulses along many nerves together. The clouds are shaped to reflect the correlational structure of what is being experienced. Such is the true language of the brain, which is well set up for it.

The brain is certainly an extraordinary structure. It is distinguished not only by the profusion of specialised cells, but also the extent of connectivity between them. The numbers alone are mind-boggling. Even the tiny brain of a fruit fly, with only a few hundred neurons, has over ten metres of 'wiring'. There are approximately 14–18 billion neurons in the human cerebral cortex, and hundreds of billions of connections. However, that it is relations, not elements, that matter is shown in the basic structural and functional organisation of the cerebral cortex, and how it has become more important in the evolution of mammals. The size of its housing in the skull is one indication. But increased folding has also achieved greater surface area and, therefore, volume. That's what has mushroomed in size in evolution from early mammals to humans (Figure 6.3).

Yet the cortex overall consists of a remarkably uniform structure consisting of six layers of cells only 3–4 mm thick. Moreover, the layers are organised as 'cortical columns', side by side. These columns exhibit abundant interconnections both within layers and between columns. And they have rich connectivity with other areas of the cortex and the rest of the brain. Estimates of numbers vary, but there are likely to be tens of millions of columns, each with up to 100 cells, achieving a total of trillions of connections (Figure 6.4).

The wiring maze makes interpretation of what's going on difficult. But something else – important for understanding intelligence – gives us

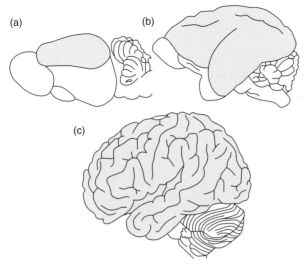

Figure 6.3 How the cerebral cortex came to dominate brain structure: (a) early mammal; (b) monkey; (c) human.

a clue. Mechanical models tend to think of processing in the brain from the bottom-up – that is, from the sensory receptors, such as the retina, to the way-stations, all converging on the cortex. That's where, it is assumed, the real business of intelligent analysis and prediction occur. However, it turns out that there are at least as many *top-down* connections conveying signals from the cortex to the 'lower' levels. For example, the retinae send signals to the lateral geniculate nuclei (LGN) in the midbrain. The LGN are supposed to be just passing on signals to the cerebral cortex for ultimate processing, but they actually receive *far more* signals from the cortex than they send to it. So what's that all about?

Moreover, such reciprocity seems to be the norm. It's the same with other sensory way-stations in the brain. Studies of rat, cat, and monkey brains show that the average send/receive connection ratio between those different regions of the cortex is close to 1, which suggests the strong role of feedback

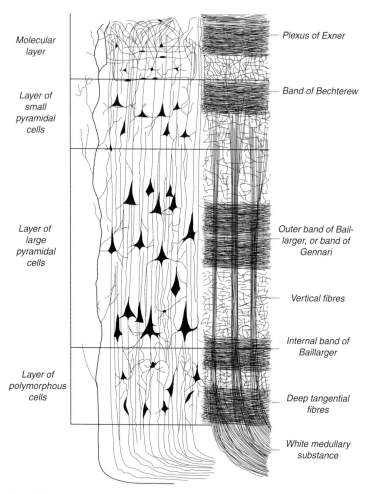

Molecular layer

Layer of small pyramidal cells

Layer of large pyramidal cells

Layer of polymorphous cells

Plexus of Exner

Band of Bechterew

Outer band of Baillarger, or band of Gennari

Vertical fibres

Internal band of Baillarger

Deep tangential fibres

White medullary substance

Figure 6.4 A representative cortical column, specially stained, on the left, to show cell bodies; and, on the right, to show cell connections. (Wikipedia, public domain).

mechanisms. Signals fed forward are all the time being reshaped by those fed back after wider 'consideration'. Such retuning and integration of bottom-up inputs with contextual information appears to be a core feature of processing in the cortex of the brain.

Sound familiar? These are multi-parallel cascades of feed-forward/feedback loops. Such loops were introduced in Chapter 3 in the context of intelligent molecular networks (and mentioned above for the retina). Here in the brain, as in those more primitive networks, an input signal is a space–time pattern of nerve impulses. It already has a certain shape or form, making a preliminary prediction of what is being sensed, like a momentary shot of a fuzzy video. This best guess is fed forward to 'higher' nodes, the cortical columns, where they are integrated with inputs from other nodes.

Those interactions provide a wider view, like standing back from a picture. As Sven Schrader and colleagues put it, 'the cortex first tries to catch the gist of the scene. The gist is then fed back as global hypothesis to influence and redirect further bottom-up processing.'

What you first thought was a blob on the horizon now turns out to be a tree. Or that smudged letter becomes decipherable in the context of the whole word. Now the first best guess looks different. In our example in the brain, a signal is fed back to the sender (in this case, the LGN) to advise an adjustment, try again, and repeat the process until a pattern that makes more sense in the context of the wider picture is obtained. The worked-up pattern now becomes a more intelligent basis for predictability and action.

There is much experimental evidence for that kind of processing. In research in 2019, neurophysiologist Mihály Bányai and his colleagues showed that identification of natural stimuli reaching the cortex critically depended on the correlational structure within it. Neuroscientist Ian Andolina and his colleagues manipulated the feedback from the cortex to the LGN in the visual processing stream. They found marked changes in the feed-forward activity.

It all happens at phenomenal speed. Signals from the retina reach the cortex within one-sixth of a second. Actual motor response (such as catching a ball) starts only a couple of hundred milliseconds later, after the loops have clarified the decision-making. A human can recognise the picture of a familiar object or person in about one-tenth of a second. Even if you've spilled coffee over part of it, or some of it has been torn away, it will take just a little longer to reconstruct. It all supports Donald Hoffman's view that, in making any sense of natural experience, we are all, in fact, 'visual geniuses', naively unaware of our rich talents.

Senses Together

Similar feed-forward/feedback coding of correlation patterns takes place in other senses. A familiar tune, a car engine, or other sound can be recognised from fragments of acoustic stimuli. In the somatosensory (tactile) domain, moving a finger over a coat button almost immediately creates an image of the whole object. From the space–time shape of correlations strong predictions can be made – such as a car approaching, so don't cross the road just yet.

The activity going on *between* different way-stations is also phenomenal. For example, of the several million axons terminating in the LGN, only about 10 per cent originate in the eyes. The rest come from several areas of cerebral cortex and a variety of subcortical regions. They are obviously doing more than just passing on features picked up in the senses. This is a general aspect of organisation in the brain. Inputs from senses become alert to each other. A long line of research on cortical neurons has shown that the receipt of inputs in sensory (e.g. visual) cortex is almost invariably accompanied by parallel or anticipatory alerts in other areas, including those associated with possible motor responses. So we can park a car with a sense of where the wheels and bumpers are even though we cannot see them.

All the time, of course, networks are being continually reconfigured, the better to anticipate future inputs, recognise and categorise them, and know what to do with them. This is learning. Scientists studying complex dynamical systems call those consequences of experience 'basins of attraction', dispersed in the connection networks. Like the spirals that form in a washbasin, it means that input samples will be drawn towards a corresponding configuration of connections, and predictions made from them, all the more expeditiously.

Cognitive Intelligence

No wonder it has been difficult to describe function-from-wiring in even the small brain of the roundworm. The world 'inside' that it makes decisions with is not a veridical reflection of the world outside. That would be pointless, and not very intelligent, because that world is ever-changing. Rather, the inside world is a construct, made up of the (often very deep) correlation patterns in experience. It permits greater insight, better predictability, and therefore more appropriate decision-making than a direct copy of the world could possibly provide.

But the construction – the squeezing of information from structure – doesn't stop there. Like groups at a convention, each having brought their own patterns of information, those emergent patterns now encounter, communicate with, and adjust and inform each other. Patterns among patterns now further emerge, transcending the originals, creating new properties in the process. The animal is now using *cognitive* intelligence, not merely input–output routines.

I have already hinted at how such intelligence in the visual system helps us 'see' far more than is 'in' direct experience. That is *visual cognition*. But it has also been explored particularly well with other senses. The identification of odours, for example, was the original distance sense, and is still of vital importance to most animals. But recognition is more than direct categorical mapping. The identification of a smell – an odour – depends on progressive condensation of correlation patterns among possibly hundreds of components, involving the usual feed-forward/feedback loops.

As cognitive scientist Ann-Sophie Barwich explains in an insightful review, that fine coffee aroma you may be sniffing is actually a combination of several hundred chemicals. None of these, in isolation, smells of coffee. (In fact one of them, on its own, has an overpowering faecal scent, but we won't go there). Moreover, Barwich reviews a number of entertaining illustrations of how, in humans, the same smelly substances can smell quite different in different contexts. That's because the result of brain processing is an abstract correlational pattern, not a discrete 'object'.

Physician Walter Freeman studied electroencephalographs (EEGs, or 'brain waves') in mice while they sniffed various substances. Each smell, he reported, produces a wave of activity in the first way-station in the brain, the olfactory bulb. This activity is rapidly fed forward to higher centres. Those centres feed back information to the first centre to clarify and stabilise the input. Freeman and colleagues suggest, then, that it is not external smells *per se* that animals respond to, at least directly: '[T]he perceptual message that is sent on into the forebrain is a construction, not the residue of a filter or a computational algorithm.'

Studies with sounds have shown, likewise, that the brain's real job is to provide 'higher' patterns, furnishing intelligent activity, not the mechanical responses of ready-made circuits. A 2015 review by neuroscientist Shaowen Bao suggests that (as with other intelligent systems) the constructions, or higher patterns, are largely 'certain statistical structures' that 'shape auditory cortical acoustic representations'. Neural circuits, he says, 'organize themselves according to the statistical structures of the sensory input'. Out of that self-organisation develops learned categorical sound perceptions laden with predictability, as in human speech sounds. Finally, working with ferrets, Victoria Bajo and Andrew King showed how neurons in the brain cortex do not respond to the acoustical properties of stimuli *per se*. They more typically respond to the acquired task-related meaning of signals – that is, their learned predictability in a wider context.

The constructed world inside will ultimately, of course, incorporate all the senses, including feelings monitoring internal states (see below) and those from nerve endings in muscles, joints, and limbs. In all these cases, the final activity pattern is now a *cognitive* construction rather than a mere neural one. It now enters a new level of interactions with wider patterns. The patterns themselves interact, and new ones emerge in the process, with staggering depths of statistical structure. The world constructed by the brain, whether it's the worm's or yours, is far richer than the one that hits its senses.

So, if you've been following so far, here's a little test. Imagine tiny, seed-sized brains being grown in a Petri dish, each cultured from a few brain cells. That's happening in a laboratory at the University of California. Could they have consciousness? A lot of people are asking that.

My take goes like this. The point of intelligent systems, especially those in the brain, is the abstraction of deep correlation patterns from an ever-changing world. From those patterns, 'inner' worlds are constructed that far exceed in depth and awareness the raw stimuli that hit our senses. That 'added value' furnishes detailed predictability (or meaning). I think that's what we can also call consciousness. Since the little brain in the lab (rather like the AI computer, or a real brain in a jar) is utterly isolated from those environmental riches it can have no consciousness. Discuss.

Of course, psychologists usually fail to see cognitive intelligence as such an emergent system. They try to map cognition directly to the level of brain networks and reduce individual differences in function to the mechanical efficiency of their physiology. So cognitive psychologists still have difficulty in describing the nature of intelligence in those networks and how it works. They tell us some of the things cognition apparently does *ad nauseum*: attention, perception, learning, memory, language, problem-solving, reasoning and thinking, even imagination, and so on. And IQ testers offer those up as 'definitions' of intelligence. But labelling is not describing, and the deeper mystery prevails.

We now should know better, and look for cognitive functions in the dynamic processing of emergent properties. I will return to them more specifically in the context of human cognition and intelligence in Chapter 8.

Experience-Dependence

The enormous pattern gathering of the brain involves continual updating and revising of network connections. But it crucially depends on correlational structure. In experimental animals it has been shown that patterned light, rather than just *any* light stimulation, appears to be required for normal development of the sensory cortex. Confining visual experience to white noise, which presents all light frequencies without the patterned input, retards development of connectivity. Likewise, random sound or noise is not sufficient for proper development of the auditory cortex. Structured sound, containing correlation patterns, is crucial.

Patterns experienced over longer periods result in a deeper configuring of networks, known as experience-dependence. Although different individuals of a species have the same complement of initial connections, their configuration in more complex networks can vary substantially between individual brains. City taxi drivers, for example, are required to develop a detailed memory of street layouts, which is strikingly reflected in the increased size of the posterior hippocampus (part of the brain involved in spatial relations). Likewise, the part of the cortex involved in finger coordination is, in violin players, expanded on the corresponding side of the brain, but not on the other. There are many other examples.

This is life-long development, as mentioned in Chapter 5: a continual strategy for dealing with a rapidly changing world. As a result, cortical connectivity is largely induced by the nature of the problem domains confronting it, rather than by predetermined architectures. That's what the brain really evolved for.

Intelligence with Feeling

Unfortunately, the mechanical-computational view of the brain and intelligence tends to neglect a place for feeling. 'Hot' emotion has often been contrasted with 'cool' reasoning, the real business of the brain. However, philosophers have often reminded us that all sensory experience is suffused with feeling. Images of desired objects, and memories and concepts of more abstract categories, such as beauty and harmony, come with feeling. So brain studies have revealed an indissoluble link between thought and emotion.

Brain activity and cognition, attention to stimuli, and what we do about them (motivation) are certainly affected by feelings. But the opposite also happens. By their nature, correlational patterns, over short or longer terms, are more or less harmonious. Their effects on cognitive states reverberate on feelings, creating ease or unease (and occasional *dis*ease). They are accompanied by floods of neural and hormonal signals around the body. Those rapidly change activities of organs, adjust physiology, recruit genes, prepare muscles for action, and even affect facial expressions. They also enhance awareness, attention, and other cognitive processes, aiding or hindering intelligence.

As a result, feelings form an integral aspect of the total network constituting the brain, and the cognitive activity it supports. Emotional salience fosters attention and, therefore, learning and memory. More importantly, in human evolution (see Chapter 7), those networks became part of an extended 'social' brain that permits humans to share feelings, to feel what another is feeling, as in empathy. That's why often the best pleasures in life are those we give to others.

In that way we each form unique 'connectomes' consolidating feelings as part of intelligent functions. The inter-relations define the self, our personalities, and individual identities. That has important implications for performances of individuals with real-life histories in real-life contexts, including testing situations and schools. How we feel influences what we make of current experience, what we think and how to act. The effects have been described as 'emotional intelligence'.

Emotional intelligence is also based on correlational patterns. For example, scenes (or artworks and photographs) having a deep correlational structure (called fractals) are judged by viewers to be most aesthetic. That appreciation is reflected in 'feel good' physiological changes in the body. Likewise, we talk about the beauties of faces, mountain scenes, and so on, as the deep structure within them stirs positive feelings. The sense of harmony makes us feel good, because it harbours predictability, from feature to feature. So (unlike any other species) we create and celebrate it. Our love of music, song and dance, games with made-up rules, and so on, all reflect how the evolved brain has turned us into pattern junkies.

Lack of integration, or disharmony, on the other hand, may produce negative feelings of frustration, disgust, fear, and so on, because of uncertainty. Either way, the dissonance is fed forward to drive cognitive searches for solutions, attempting to integrate one set of patterns with others, and construct a novel course of action. Results are fed back to test against feelings, and further results fed forward. In those loops are spun the world of emotional intelligence. Little wonder that intense feelings are often viewed as essential ingredients in rich cognition, constructive action, and inspired creativity. Conversely, need for structure and pattern also means being prone to mythology and ideology (of which, more in Chapter 8). It all explains, however, why a computer could never be a substitute for a real brain in a real body in a social world.

MRI: Seeing Intelligence?

In spite of the parallel connectivity and feed-forward/feedback loops just described, the search for simple maps, from genes to brain 'wiring', or from wiring to cognitive ability, persists. The dream of being able to attribute individual differences in intelligence to (presumed immutable) differences in brains or brain parts continues. It has a long history. Victorian scientists tried to attribute intelligence differences to brain size and invented craniometry. Measures included simple head circumference in living subjects. Or they filled the crania of the dead with lead shot, it's weight then used as an index of brain volume. Differences between social classes, and between sexes, were duly reported as proof of differences in intelligence. In the British colonies, equally reassuring conclusions about the brains of different 'races' were reached. Even today, claims are being made about brain size and intelligence, with similar conclusions.

These efforts have been boosted recently by the use of MRI scans. The process, the data produced, and interpretations of them are extremely technical and indirect, but I will try to simplify. It involves sliding an individual or individual's head into an enclosed cylinder, with instructions issued through internal transmitters. The scan machine creates a magnetic field in the target tissue, thus agitating protons in the atoms within it. When the magnetic field is turned off, the protons stop jiggling. In doing so they give off an electrical signal that can be measured. The signal strength varies, depending on the density of the tissues. So the scan can distinguish, for example, between brain and bone (skull); or between grey matter (such as densely packed neurons) and white matter (more dispersed axons sheathed in fatty tissue). This 'structural' MRI has been mainly used for measuring brain size or aspects of brain structure, such as specific nerve tracts or regions. A number of studies using it have suggested correlations of 0.2–0.4 between IQ and brain size. These values have been widely accepted but also challenged.

Another approach, functional MRI (fMRI), has been used to detect changes in brain tissues while getting the individual to perform cognitive tasks, such as those in IQ tests. It relies on the increased blood flow to active parts of the brain. The blood carries more oxygen, again producing varying signals. These are taken as proxies for brain activity on the presumption that blood is being sent there to support the mental activity.

Impressive coloured pictures of parts of the brain 'lighting up' during activation are now familiar to anyone who reads newspapers or magazines. Big claims have been made about how they reveal relations between brain size, surface area of the cortex, thickness of nerve tracts, or sizes of specific regions, and differences in IQ. Studies are described as brain-wide association studies (BWAS), analogous with the gene-wide association studies (GWAS) described in Chapter 2. Inevitably, attempts are also being made to correlate those correlations with genomic sequencing differences (see Chapter 2), thus perpetuating the tacit model:

Genetic differences → brain differences→ intelligence differences.

In neuroscience generally, and in medicine, there is no doubt that structural MRI scans have been a game-changer. Fine anatomical details can be described at microscopic levels, a boon to diagnostics. But real problems start when psychologists think that fMRI scans take us inside the 'black box' and discover how it relates to intelligence, and individual differences in it. As with the genome sequencing studies, there is abundant scope for spurious correlations. Take size first. Unless we adopt the crudest of mechanical models there is no biological reason why (within a species) brain size (or that of any organ) should be directly correlated with function. There are huge differences in brain sizes among humans, mostly between 1,000 and 1,500 cubic centimetres. They exist without obvious differences in everyday cognitive functions. Men's brains are about 10 per cent bigger than women's, on average, without clear differences in intelligence.

More significantly, a vast range of childhood and adult experiences have effects on both brain size and test performances. Take, for example, the Romanian adopted children studied by psychiatrist Michael Rutter and colleagues. Prior to adoption they had experienced enormous stress in overcrowded and neglectful care homes. That was associated with much-reduced brain volume in adulthood, and in proportion to duration of stress.

Also, stress in pregnancy or early childhood, malnutrition, exposure to toxic substances, drugs, and so on may be reflected in both brain size and test performances. Even mothers' stress prior to pregnancy may affect brain size in their children, without necessarily affecting cognitive ability. These experiences vary across different social classes, which also carry different (but probably irrelevant) gene variants. And social classes, for various reasons, vary in IQ. So, again, scope for spurious correlations is enormous.

Such factors were noted in a major critique in the *Journal of the American Medical Association* in 2020, by Daniel Weinberger and Eugenia Radulescu. Noting that MRIs do not directly measure the brain, but tiny magnetic changes agitated within it, they say:

> Substantial variation in brain dimensions as measured on MRI can be associated with variation in water content, tissue perfusion, body weight, cholesterol levels, imperceptible head motion, endogenous steroid levels, time of day, and even exercise and mental activities. Because many of these confounders tend to segregate with the study population, the potential for misattribution of cause is substantial.

So the method is prone to spurious and unreliable correlations. But that is compounded in fMRIs by another overarching problem. However seductive those colourful pictures, they are difficult to interpret. In his book *Innate*, Kevin Mitchell adopts a strong wiring-determined basis for IQ differences. But he also says that deciphering the scans needs 'a lot of unglamorous statistics to extract the signal from both the noise and the background activity'. The fact is that differences in signals, over background fluctuations, especially in the cognitive tasks, are usually tiny, often less than 2 per cent. To reach statistical significance, researchers typically must average many trials of the same task from many different individuals. That introduces more variation. More circumspect researchers were therefore not surprised to read a major report in *Nature* in May 2020, in which 70 independent teams were asked to analyse the same scans, and substantial inconsistency in interpretation transpired.

In another 2020 study published in *Psychological Science*, it was also found that overall reliability across a number of studies was poor. But the researchers further examined results in which participants were tested and then retested. The test–retest reliabilities of brain activities across 11 common fMRI tasks were weak. The researchers concluded that 'these findings demonstrate that common task-fMRI measures are not currently suitable for brain biomarker discovery or for individual-differences research'. Commenting on these inconsistencies, neuroscientist Ahmad Hariri reminds us that the level of activity for any given person probably won't be the same twice and found that 'the correlation between one scan and a second is not even fair, it's poor' – task-based fMRI in its current form can't tell you what an individual's brain activation will look like from one test to the next.

As with the genetic studies, there are also doubts about the quality of 'intelligence' testing. One popular test, for example, claims to measure individuals' 'executive functions' in four minutes! But the fundamental problem is the mechanical, 'power-driven' model of both brain and intelligence underpinning such studies. It is reminiscent of the failure to map function to brain wiring, or 'atlas', in even the simple brain of the roundworm, as described in Chapter 4.

Regarding more advanced brains, network scientist Mehraveh Salehi and her colleagues argued in their 2020 review, that 'there remains an underlying assumption that such an atlas exists', although 'no single functional atlas has emerged as the dominant atlas to date'. The title of their paper is 'There is no single functional atlas *even for a single individual*' (my emphasis). Instead, their research shows (as I've just tried to describe here), 'that functional atlases reconfigure substantially and in a meaningful manner, according to brain state'. This means that what is happening locally depends on the intelligent system of brain and cognition as a whole, and its experience-dependence in the current social context. The 'state' of the brain's intelligent system may arise in a bony cranium, but certainly not in an isolated box. It emerges from interactions in nerve networks, themselves in continual interaction with physiology, in continual interaction with metabolic and epigenetic processes, and continual learning at every level. To say that intelligence is somehow 'in' the brain is to miss so much of its truly dynamic function.

7 Becoming Human

So far I have tried to show how intelligence evolved at different levels according to the complexity of the environments faced. We have just seen how the breakthrough to cognitive intelligence emerged from the chatter between neurons in large networks. In this chapter, I show how human evolution involved another, even more stunning, breakthrough in a way not fully appreciated but fully consistent with biological principles. As with intelligent systems generally, it emerged from social interaction at a number of levels, not lucky genetic accidents.

This is an important point because it is usually put by scientists – and accepted by the general public – that competing individuals and natural selection somehow gave us smart brains and better intelligence. Eventually, that superior intelligence led humans to realise the good sense in cooperating to some extent. But it remains up to each individual to negotiate that social life as a means for serving personal ends, using whatever cunning he or she can muster. That is the kind of story, and the implied nature of intelligence, that has been put forward by evolutionary psychologists for most of the last century.

The reality, though, is the other way around. It was the success of cooperation that founded the more complex intelligent systems we all have. As described in Chapters 3 and 4, intelligent life was social almost from the start. The profusion of forms, integrated functions, and sheer complexity of multicellular organisms, could not have arisen otherwise. By missing that reality, we have been missing so much in understanding, not just human intelligence, but also our relations with each other and the rest of the world. This chapter explores that theme in evolution, and shows how it explains the uniqueness of humans.

Swarm Intelligence

A striking case is that of social insects such as ants and bees. So complex and intense are their social lives that socio-biologists have drawn parallels with human intelligence. Using the term 'swarm intelligence', the organisation of their colonies has even been described as like a little brain. A 2014 article by neuroscientist Carrie Arnold, in the journal *Nautilus*, is even titled 'Ants swarm like brains think'.

Ant colonies have been the subject of much fascinating research. The challenging question has concerned how their collective behaviour can be so well coordinated. It obviously requires a system of communication. Some of that is through direct contact via antennae, legs, and mouthparts, as well as visual motion. But most is through a dozen or so chemical messages called 'pheromones' laid by individuals and picked up through chemical senses by others. Some pheromones mark trails to food sources, some broadcast alarms, while others signal 'burrow here' for nest-building. The signals can quickly summon thousands of ants, not as a disorganised mass, but in coordinated divisions of labour. That suggests the communication must be structured in some way. It's like the 'swarm-ing' of slime moulds, mentioned in Chapter 4, but on a higher level, and with even more dramatic changes to the development of individual forms.

As with signalling networks in the cell, or morphogens in development, it is all self-organised, with no overall controller. Communication dynamics emerge as rapid feed-forward/feedback loops between individuals and the wider group. Individual action (feed-forward signal) is conditioned by the wider pattern of social actions. The feedback from that reshapes individual actions accordingly. Individually, ants have only around a quarter of a million neurons each, but the limited cognitive capacity within brains is greatly amplified through the emerging patterns of behaviour between them. Those obtain higher statistical patterns that take individuals beyond the information given. Even for an ant it's a complex, changing world. Studies of swarm intelligence in honeybees have made similar points.

Much of that adaptability in social insects is obtained through morphological (body) and physiological specialisation, as well as behaviour. Developmental plasticity creates different castes with distinct tasks, such as reproduction, foraging, defence, and nest maintenance. Individuals belonging to different social castes show distinct molecular, physical, and behavioural tendencies, usually established at the larval stage. It is reminiscent of the way that different cells are formed in the multicellular organism, though now at the higher level of combined individuals. That obviously furnished new levels of adaptability. But rather than wholesale bodily and metabolic specialisation, its further evolution became based primarily on behaviour involving bigger brains. That, too, went through different levels of complexity.

Shoals, Flocks, and Herds

Fish in shoals, birds in flocks, and ungulates in herds have individually much bigger brains and cognitive systems than ants. But their social intelligence seems more shallow (some people call it herd stupidity). That probably reflects its more limited function, thought to be mainly predator avoidance, such as increased awareness and the heaving, swerving group movement that causes confusion in attackers. However, large herds can include some complex relations within them. For example, they can form monogamous or polygamous relations, or exist as stable mixed-sex herds. Such differences have been shown to correlate with average brain size, itself usually taken to be an index of intelligence in a species.

Some fish and birds often display rapid, collective movements that seem to be extremely well synchronised and coordinated. The famous 'murmurations' of starlings have been particularly well researched. Rapid twists and turns occur without collisions, and without obvious executive or supervisory agents. Experiments with sonar technology have shown how the group choreography is achieved by responses in individuals interacting with the structural dynamics emerging in the group as a whole. It seems to depend on extremely rapid feed-forward/feedback loops. And they are very effective in confusing and dodging an attacking hawk or falcon.

Again, ecological conditions seem to have conditioned social interaction. That, in turn, influences the form of intelligence. So let's explore that theme further.

Mammal Intelligence

Among mammals, brain size is taken as a rough index of intelligence, but it varies enormously according to the environmental conditions they live with. Brain sizes increase with body size as more tissue, especially muscle, demands more innervation. Increases are also related to behaviour, including diet. Cats have bigger brains than rats and other rodents, in relation to body size, perhaps because they hunt for food. Primates (lemurs, monkeys, and apes) may have evolved bigger brains for distance vision, finer visual discrimination, and digital dexterity, as in picking leaves and fruit from trees. Those that catch and eat insects, for example, have still bigger brains.

Many mammals became social for the advantages it affords in food foraging and defence against predators. It is assumed that living in groups itself demands complexity of intelligence and bigger brains for managing complex relational information. With respect to primates in particular it is referred to as the 'social brain hypothesis'. For example, primatologist Robin Dunbar has argued that when the size of a social group increases, the number of different relationships in the group may increase. So primate social life has been proposed as a useful model for the origins of human intelligence.

The definitions of 'complexity' and 'social', however, may seem rather shallow. In their book *Thinking Big: How the Evolution of Social Life Made Us Human*, Dunbar and colleagues allude to 'the subtleties of how individuals interact with each other' in pre-human primates. But their emphasis is on strategies and deceptions through which individuals compete for individual advantage. It involves a degree of 'bonding', 'mind reading', and so on, as ways of gaining advantage over others. Otherwise 'interaction' is tit-for-tat, with cooperation as a kind of fortuitous and occasional side-effect. Other accounts of such social life even seem to echo Donald Trump's *The Art of the Deal*, with its emphasis on branding, marketing, and publicity.

So connections between primate social life and evolving cognitive intelligence remain unclear. Correlations between group size and brain size have been reported, but the evidence has been disputed. There is no necessary relation between group size and complexity of relations within them, anyway. Think of those vast herds of wildebeests, swarms of locusts, and so on. There are other reasons for doubting that we might find 'what made us human' in the behaviour of primates, and I will return to that in a moment.

Cooperative Hunting

For animals that hunt for a living, the environment is much more complex than it is for monkeys and apes, both physically and socially. Prey, after all, are not passive targets like leaves and tree fruits. They move rapidly and erratically against ever-changing backgrounds. That presents enormous challenges to perception, cognition, and behaviour. That is the case even for animals that hunt alone, even though they're limited to prey smaller than themselves. That limitation has been overcome in species that cooperate in tracking and capturing bigger prey. Your cat may catch a mouse or a bird, but it would take several cats acting cooperatively to catch something of their own size or even bigger.

Occasional group hunting has been reported in species that normally forage or capture prey alone. These include some fish, some birds, other mammals, and chimpanzees. It is not clear, however, whether that amounts to opportunistic 'lucky strikes', involving small prey and demanding little extra cognitive ability. However, cooperative hunting is clearly a systematic way of life in a number of species of wild dogs and one wild cat (the lion). And it involves a further leap in effective environmental complexity.

Try to think about a group of animals acting jointly in such a dynamic activity, and about what goes on in their cognitive systems. A *shared* picture of the target and its surround, is required, of course. But the target is moving rapidly, in different and constantly changing directions. So the picture 'in mind' has to be just as rapidly updated, perhaps at intervals of fractions of a second. In addition, each individual in the group is getting the picture from different angles and distances. Moreover, if individuals are to coordinate their actions they must continually relate their personal pictures to the global picture of the group, all in relation to the target. They must also be able to switch roles, and therefore viewpoints, creatively and rapidly. Then individual motor responses need to be globally coordinated in some sort of shared and moving tableau. Finally, it means coordinating self-control of feelings, including self-restraint, with those of the group as a whole.

Among such cooperative mammals, African hunting dogs have been well studied for their habit of running down prey through divisions of labour. Success depends on surrounding the prey, strategic delays, flanking and ambush manoeuvres, and other tactics of organisation. Similar patterns have been studied in wolves and lions.

But is it reflected in brain size? The few comparative data available are inconclusive. Spotted hyaenas hunt cooperatively and have larger brains and expanded frontal cortices compared with other hyaenas that hunt alone. In any case, increased folding of the cerebral cortex may have been more critical than sheer size. It may be worth noting that today's pet dogs have brains about 30 per cent smaller than those of their coopera-tive wolf ancestors, even allowing for differences in body size! It is also worth mentioning that there would have been limits to increasing brain size in four-legged animals chasing prey. It would have been difficult to carry heavier skulls, jaws, and teeth at the end of an extended neck. Perhaps substantial increases in brain size would have only been possible in an upright, bipedal species with the bigger head balanced on a vertical spine.

Interestingly, in his *Origin of Species* (1859), Charles Darwin noted that individual struggle has been replaced by cooperation in many animal spe-cies. Later, in the *Descent of Man* (1871), he pointed out how that creates the conditions for the evolution of greater 'intellectual faculties'. He suggested that the fittest are not those with the greatest *individual* strength or cunning, but those that learn mutual support for the benefit of the group as a whole. In doing so, he was pre-figuring the historical chasm in theorising about intelli-gence that has survived him. The idea of human intelligence as a form of personal 'fitness' continues to dominate IQ theory. It also survives in attempts to reconcile human intelligence with that of our ape ancestors. On that point it's worth backtracking a little to now ask how well other primates actually cooperate.

Cooperative Apes?

The idea that primates, generally, present a good model for understanding human intelligence is widespread. They certainly have complex social lives in the sense of group living, tit-for-tat reciprocity, grooming, food sharing, and so on. They also engage in much observational and trial-and-error learning. Yet even our nearest cousins – chimps, gorillas, and orangutans – are not very cooperative in the sense just described. Monkeys and apes rarely help group members other than close family, and joint action and teaching are also rare. There is little evidence, even among chimpanzees, of agreement to share or of reciprocation, and they generally feed alone. And groups are not very cohesive. Rather, temporary subgroupings called parties come together and separate throughout the day.

Occasional cooperative hunting has been reported in chimps, mainly in capturing monkeys. But it appears to be opportunistic rather than a stable habit, happening when the likelihood of a capture appears high. Also, the prey tend to be small, mostly young monkeys. The main strategy consists of one member of the party rushing the prey while others block escape routes. That requires some anticipation of movements of the 'driver' it seems. But only rarely does it involve anticipating the actions of other party members as a whole.

Otherwise, cooperation in primates consists of temporary alliances within the group, competing with other alliances. These lack what has been called 'shared intentionality'. As psychologist Michael Tomasello put it in his book, *A Natural History of Human Thinking*, chimps do not self-monitor, nor align their own thinking with that of the group as a whole. Communication, vocal or gestural, consists of stereotyped signals, almost always to request, warn, or dictate, rather than as a means of joint action. After years of making comparisons, Tomasello says that humans are evolved for collaboration in a way that apes are not. So we probably need to think again about the real origins of human intelligence.

Human Evolution

In stark contrast, there is little doubt that even the early ancestors of humans were cooperative hunters as a significant part of their way of life. Numerous excavations at fossil sites have shown how it all started in Africa, in times of unprecedented ecological challenges around seven million years ago. The general story is that the climate dried, forests thinned, and former forest-dwellers were forced onto the forest margins and open savannah. There they faced unreliable food supplies and the need to explore new food sources across wider ranges, with exposure to large predators, and so on. But there is still much debate about it.

Up to about four or five million years ago, several lineages (species) of pre-humans probably co-existed, with brains still about the size of today's chimpanzees (340–360 cubic centimetres, compared with an average of 1,400 in modern humans). They had split from a common human–ape ancestor several million years previously. Excavations at home sites suggests that between 4.5 and 2.0 million years ago our ancestors were then living in small groups of 20–30 individuals, possibly on lake margins or river flood-plains. Fossils indicate that they had evolved bipedalism (walking upright), perhaps for greater vigilance over tall grass or pursuit running. That also seems to have freed their hands for tool-making and -use. Remains of animal bones around those fossils also suggest the targeting of large prey and butchering with crude stone choppers. Brain size had increased to about 450–500 cubic centimetres.

From two million years ago, with further climate and habitat change, at least three species of our own lineage (*Homo*) emerged. They had larger body sizes, but lighter skeletons and skulls, further suggesting pursuit running. Smaller teeth and jaws also indicate less reliance on tough vegetable matter in the diet. Excavation of sites also suggests living in larger groups, with cooperative hunting of large game as a key activity. Brain size had increased some 30 per cent to around 650 cubic centimetres.

Shortly afterwards, the scene became dominated by a new species, *Homo erectus*, with bigger brains reaching around 1,200 cubic centimetres by 200,000 years ago. Migrating out of Africa, that lineage encountered harsher climates, uncertain food supplies, fierce predators like sabre tooth tigers, and huge woolly mammoths. But intelligent systems rose to the challenge. They invented fire, cooking, and warm clothing, lived in seasonal home bases, and engaged in long-distance hunting strategies for large game.

Their production of tools also stands out. The earlier *Homo* sites are associated with crude stone flakes, rounded hammer stones, and possible stone weapons. *Homo erectus* produced more sophisticated, task-specific hand axes, cutting flints, and others, all demanding imagination, dexterity, and great hand–eye coordination. The uniformity of tool shape also suggests a group design, or production with others 'in mind'. They have been found around the remains of very large prey (elephant, bison, and so on). That suggests very advanced cooperative hunting skills.

The famous Neanderthals and their cousins lived in Europe from about 400,000 years ago. They were confronted with even more harsh climatic and ecological circumstances, including several ice ages. Sites all over Europe and parts of Asia also suggest new methods for the systematic production of flakes and blades, as well as wooden spears, with more sophisticated and stereotyped shapes. That implies the sharing of perceptions and cognitions as mentioned earlier, as well as rules for group behaviour and a system of communication more sophisticated than the 30 or so fixed signals of the chimpanzee. And these were still pre-modern-humans.

Homo sapiens

Sometime around 200,000 years ago (there is still uncertainty), anatomically modern *Homo sapiens* originated in Africa and started to fan out in all directions. They reached Asia and Europe perhaps 100,000 years ago, eventually replacing the Neanderthals and their cousins that had been there for some time. They appear to have existed in large social bands, with possible alliances between them, and extremely successful social hunting of large game. That also suggests intimate knowledge of the prey, their typical behaviour patterns, and of local and wider ecology, while suffering exposure to predators, weather patterns, and so on.

Living sites have also revealed vast improvements in material culture. The tools of *Homo erectus* (and the Neanderthals) had remained fairly

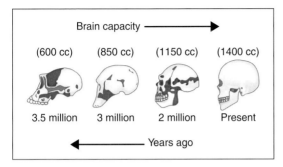

Figure 7.1   Increasing brain sizes from early to modern *Homo* (https://dragonflyissuesi nevolution13.wikia.org, posted by Katejn aka Kate Nordyke, Creative Commons licence).

stereotyped for over a million years. The arrival of *Homo sapiens*, however, is marked by a spectacular creativity and variability of style. Apart from stonework, the toolbox includes a complex bone technology and multiple-faceted missile heads, harpoons, pointed spears, and bows and arrows. The distribution of these, and of artefacts like perforated seashells and bone ornaments, also suggests trading between groups (the importance of which, for intelligence, I return to below).

Finally, fossil skulls from that period indicate a huge increment of brain expansion, reaching the modern human average of 1,400 cubic centimetres (Figure 7.1). That is about three times bigger than the average for chimpanzee brain, in relation to body size. And that obscures a vast increase in folding of the cerebral cortex, with increased functional volume – a quite phenomenal transformation of a bodily organ over a relatively short evolutionary time. It's as if evolutionary forces had created a rich, and previously unsurpassed, form of intelligent adaptability (Figure 7.2). What could it have been?

Fit for Social Life

Darwin's theory of gradual evolution naturally inclines us to emphasise the continuities between human and non-human intelligence. Cognitive differences have been downplayed as ones 'of degree and not of kind' (as Darwin

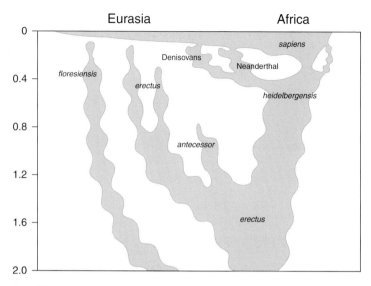

Figure 7.2   Very quickly, from around 200,000 years ago, the modern human intelligence system eclipsed antecedents. Vertical axis is in millions of years before present (from Wikipedia licensed under Creative Commons. Original from Chris Stringers' hypothesis of the family tree of genus Homo, published in Stringer, C. (2012). 'What makes a modern human'. Nature 485 (7396): 33–35. DOI:10.1038/485033a).

put it). Many theorists have warned against a 'sterile searching for a cognitive Rubicon' between apes and humans. Looking at the evolution of intelligent *systems*, though, indicates that many such leaps *have* occurred: from single cells to multicellular organisms; from local cell signalling to body-wide physiology; from those to behaviour regulated by brains and then cognitive systems. Each 'social' transition entailed significant transformation of antecedents. Even the getting together of slime moulds involved wholesale reconfiguration of the metabolic networks of prior individuals. Yet they have all occurred with seamless biological continuity. So I am hoping to describe how the biggest leap of all – to human intelligence – is perfectly in keeping with evolutionary biology, while telling us how much *is* spectacularly different from its antecedents.

As described above, conditions of survival for early humans meant life was extremely perilous. They would have experienced periods of intense biological selection, meaning severe elimination of the less fit.

But what they had to be 'fit' for was not those hazards and challenges in a direct sense. Rather, they were dealt with collectively. What they had to be *primarily* fit for was the ability to participate fully in a cooperative social life. That social world is vastly more complex than the physical world, as we have seen, and more so than the social world of monkeys and apes. That has made the biology of humans unique in many ways.

The demands of that social life, dealing with such harsh conditions, meant passing through genetic 'bottlenecks' – so harsh indeed, that it is thought that, at various times, there may have been only a few thousand of this emerging species surviving. One result is the way that humans are genetically remarkably alike, sharing at least 99 per cent of our genes around the world.

That doesn't mean that there is no genetic diversity in humans. Due to natural selection, members of any species can be genetically very alike in crucial traits (see Chapter 3), while remaining highly variant in traits of lesser importance. It's the latter variants that delight, but often confuse, those involved in DNA sequencing studies, as described in Chapter 2 (and also mislead racists, as I will describe in Chapter 8). Also bear in mind that genes are resources for development and survival, not programmes, and they can be used in alternative ways. What they were resources for in evolving humans was a new, social, way of dealing with the world. The emergent intelligent system became a new 'method', on a new level, for creating both variation and adaptation on a scale far outstripping all others. Let us now have a look at what that 'method' consisted of; how that complexity with diversity has come about; and how it manifested itself in cognitive abilities and intelligence.

The Social Brain

The brain tripled in size in evolution from apes to humans. But nearly all of that occurred in a vast neocortex, the part of the brain conventionally thought of as dealing with 'higher-order' cognitive functions. In humans, 90 per cent of the cerebral cortex and 76 per cent of the entire brain is neocortex. Most significantly, though, nearly all of it consists of a vast replication of those cortical columns already evolved in ancestral mammals (see Chapter 6).

What could they be for? Consider lifting and moving a table or a cupboard with a friend. You will become aware of the natural correlations between forces of mass, gravity, shape, and friction. But those all become conditioned by the (perhaps unpredictable) interactions with your partner. Each has now to take account of that new complexity of forces in order for the joint action to become coordinated. In addition, of course, all these forces have to be geared to an overall, *shared* conception of your joint purpose. Such depth of pattern isn't even remotely experienced in the social interactions of non-cooperating animals.

That's what those extra cortical columns in a hugely expanded brain are for: to foster the new emergent layer of coordination *between* brains. In them, the familiar feed-forward/feedback system became more important than ever. The behaviour (including verbal and other communication) of individuals becomes feed-forward information to others in a group. *Their* cognitions produce tentative responses (movement, gesture, or speech) as feedback. At first (as in moving an object together) there will be little coordination. But rapid back and forth interaction between the cognitive and social levels leads to emergence of an abstract, but shared, plan.

Philosopher-psychologists have, for centuries, sensed that 'something' emerges between cooperating minds that is more than the sum of its parts. Sometimes it has been called 'group mind' or, more recently, 'collective intelligence'. In rather nebulous forms, the subject has cropped up in sociology, psychology, business studies, computer studies, and so on. Researchers following individuals solving problems collectively tend to confirm a 'group' advantage. But the processes behind it have remained unclear.

As with other levels of intelligence, I see it as more than a mere aggregation of individual contributions. It is a dynamic interactive process of feed-forward /feedback loops, now with emergent patterns between brains, not merely within them. The result is another level of predictability. The patterns and their predictability transcend the contributions of any individual while

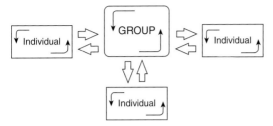

Figure 7.3   Feed-forward/feedback loops between cooperating individuals result in an emergent level of intelligence.

feeding back to enhance and extend them (Figure 7.3). What is in the 'box' are shared patterns forming the rules of cooperation, just as the rules of grammar in speech are the emerged patterns of sharing of sounds.

Many attempts are currently being made to adequately describe the very real, but invisible, structures between cooperating individuals. Some have referred to 'hyperbrain networks'. Others have referred to a 'super-brain', the 'invisible social brain', 'distributed' social cognition, or 'interthinking'. The point is that brain-to-brain coupling constrains and shapes the actions of each individual. Emergent rules foster complex joint behaviours that could not have emerged in isolation. It has had profound and revolutionary ramifications in what we call human culture.

Culture

There have been many attempts to 'bridge the gap' to humans by looking for some presence of culture in other species. The efforts have been focused, for example, on the discovery that some primates can use sticks or stones as simple tools, and they can copy their use from one another. Chimps copy others using sticks to dip for termites, or a stone to crack a nut. Monkeys can copy their parents' trick of washing potatoes on the seashore. The inference has been, in effect, to say 'look, other primates have culture – we're not that different after all'.

However, that's like comparing the 'quorum sensing' between slime moulds (see Chapter 4) with the true physiology in multicellular organisms. Mere copying of behaviours from one another is not human culture. 'Learning from' is not the same as 'learning with'. It's like comparing human speech – jointly created abstract rules – with the mere mimicking of a parrot. Human culture is not merely 'transmitted', but jointly cultivated. It then becomes manifest in many tangible and intangible forms, as 'cultural tools'. This is evident even in stone-age tool-making. By a 150,000 years ago, a vast range of technological tools were being fashioned for shared use. Such cultural effervescence has dominated human history ever since.

Human language probably soon evolved as a unique device for coordinating thoughts and feelings in joint perception and joint action. But there are simpler ways of doing that, too. Conventions, such as head nods and finger pointing, indicate what to jointly attend to. End goals and routes to it are shared in plans and maps, even those drawn in the sand. Other gestures monitor and adjust progress. These have all been called 'cultural tools'. Intelligent division of labour (as in moving an object together) is also a cultural tool. Queuing, or turn-taking, is another. Various other inventions for thought sharing (e.g. number and writing systems) have also emerged. More abstract are sets of rules and conventions governing rights and responsibilities in the group as a whole: in reproduction and parenting; in arrangements for sharing fruits of joint activities; as ideologies for ordering of people into social classes; expectations for controlling and sharing feelings; and so on.

Many cultural tools become shared in tangible representations called symbols. They include totems, flags, forms of dress, trophies, emblems, songs, slogans, and even particular individuals, such as priests and leaders. They enshrine, in overt form, deeper patterns of relations, as in group identity, shared understandings, and so on. They reinforce feelings of security and predictability. Indeed, some authors have tried to distinguish human intelligence by describing us as a unique 'symbolic species'. As such, symbolic tools are widely used to arouse relations and associated feelings. Sadly, they are also sometimes misused in attempts to resurrect relations that no longer exist, as in symbols of empires and conquests past. The effect is to by-pass intelligent, critical thinking.

Collections of cultural tools are what comprise a human culture. But the patterns are neither fixed in time nor necessarily confined to each group. They can merge and interact, fostering even wider possibilities for dealing with the world, and that seems to have been happening for a long time. Excavations of sites over 200,000 years old have discovered that some materials for tool-making came from far distant sources. That suggests that humans living then had already developed trade networks.

The significance of that for intelligence amounts to another level of demands on cognition – another layer of feed-forward/feedback loops for boosting intelligence. All those demands for inter-group culture seem to offer the best explanation for the huge increase in brain size, especially in the numbers of those cortical columns in the brain's neocortex. The expansion of connections with emotional centres of the brain (see Chapter 6) and sharing of feelings also explains why humans are often so eager to help others, even total strangers. It makes the helpers feel better, too.

But what further resilience and creativity it yielded! Contact *between* cultures has probably been vital to the survival and development of evolving humans. The more contact the groups had, the more innovative their technologies and cultures became. That's how they managed to evolve and journey across the earth, learning from each other and adapting the world to themselves, rather than vice versa.

Cultured Intelligence

In evolution's latest leap, human cognition has become fashioned by its socio-cultural tools, just as the activities of neurons are fashioned by the global activity of networks, or the behaviour of ants is fashioned by the emergent intelligence of the swarm. We can get some sense of that in the way that even a crude stone hammer or hand axe shapes patterns of movement in our joints and limbs. Likewise for today's more sophisticated wrenches, drills, or machines. They all significantly extend our otherwise limited manual capabilities.

Other cultural tools, however, work as *psychological* tools. By shaping human cognitive capabilities, they hugely extend, amplify, and diversify them. That means thinking about human intelligence, and individual differences in it, in quite a different way: horsepower in engines, or computational capacity in digital processors, are really hopeless analogies. A few illustrations may help.

Incorporation into a Social World

From the first moments of birth, human infants meet their worlds through and with other people. That means with cultural tools. In pioneering research in the 1970s, psychologist Jerome Bruner and others observed how the infant's gestures and movements are fed forward to observant adults. Based on adults' own cultural developments the infants are thus imputed with intentions, desires, and feelings. That becomes the feedback that does much to shape infant cognition and future responses. By four months old, infants can register correlational patterns in social interactions and use them to generate expectancies (predictions) from and with carers. This is what is called 'intersubjectivity', and it transforms individual intelligence.

It is in this way that the infant becomes incorporated into a structured social world. For example, just moments after giving birth, parents are told the infant's sex. Imputed predispositions then give rise to gender categorisation with deep consequences for individual psychology. But even physical objects become parts of patterns of social relations. At first the infant handles a spoon, say, as he or she would any natural object. But this handling becomes slowly, but radically, reorganised by adult feedback to conform to more specific social uses such as feeding. Again, a cultural tool transforms and extends individual cognitions.

In countless other ways, including rules for behaviour, reading, writing, and so on, child development consists of the progressive internalisation of cultural tools that also shape their intelligence. It is through such processes that humans come to think and act. From toilet training to becoming an airline pilot, a scientist, or a bus driver, socially devised tools become individual cognitive tools.

Thinking and Reasoning

Above all else, it is assumed, human intelligence is expressed in the thinking or reasoning (i.e. productive thinking) of individuals. Indeed, items in IQ tests tend to be invented to reflect such assumptions. Hence the almost reverential respect for analogies, matrices, and so on, as described in Chapter 1. It assumes reasoning to be based on 'built-in' computational processes that vary in strength or power across individuals.

In keeping with that view, some logicians, philosophers, and cognitive psychologists have tried to reduce human thinking to fixed, law-like processes 'in the head'. But doing so hasn't been straightforward. Researchers have been puzzled that individuals have some difficulty with problems like:

All *A*s are *B*s.
Are all *B*s *A*s?

But the difficulties evaporate when essentially the same problems are presented in familiar contexts, such as:

All humans are mammals.
Are all mammals humans?

Some psychologists might argue that the first of those is a better test of intelligence because it relies on more 'abstract' thinking. That ignores the way that the abstract is itself related to experience. Individuals can be readily trained on them. As cross-cultural psychologist Sylvia Scribner pointed out, the puzzles involve reaching foregone conclusions from otherwise meaningless premises. She suggests that much classroom learning in schools is like that, and that's why schoolchildren become better at them, as her research in developing countries showed.

As with all logical reasoning, what really matters is how it relates to real-life contexts. As educational psychologist Robert Glaser put it, *effective* thinking is always associated with 'the conditions and constraints of its use'. Even the archetypal case of mathematics involves structures that are abstract relations or patterns from real experience. In contrast, as cognitive scientists Hugo Mercier and Dan Sperber say in their book, *The Enigma of Reason*, 'Logic, rather than a basis for reasoning, is a formalised system developed by logicians that has little connection to actual human reasoning.'

That explains the problem encountered by psychologist Daniel Kahneman in his best-seller, *Thinking Fast and Slow*. He describes how so many people fail seemingly simple 'logical' tasks in the laboratory. Indeed, even people with high IQs can make silly mistakes on little tests such as the following:

> A bat and ball cost a dollar and ten cents. The bat costs a dollar more than the ball. How much does the ball cost?

Most people confidently blurt out that the ball costs ten cents, which is the wrong answer. A little reflection should tell you that the ball costs five cents.

Kahneman says the difficulty stems from people having *two* systems of cognition. One provides immediate inferences and intuitions about situations. The other scrutinises their logical validity in terms of the kind of abstract logic just mentioned. But it's a classical mechanical-computational model that does not really explain the origins and creativity of human social cognition. The discomfort is revealed most when we ask where did these systems come from, and how did they arise or evolve? Kahneman's answer is to kick the issue into psychology's familiar long grass: they are 'innate', he says, we are 'born with them'. Which of course is no answer at all. I suspect that is the cost of encapsulating human intelligence as individual, mechanical processes, instead of the feed-forward/feedback dialogue between the cultural and individual levels.

Researchers studying creative human intelligence understand the importance of that dialogue. Psychologist Nathalie Bonnardel and colleagues study the reasoning process in real problem-solving, as in product design. It is interesting how they use terms like 'bottom up and top down' or '*reflective conversation* between the designer and external representations'. They also describe how creativity in design 'is based on the interaction between a person and the environment, and is intrinsically related to human activity with and within the world'.

Language

It is unfortunate that, since the 1950s, language has been modelled, much like cognition in general, as a 'computational system' based on built-in rules. Psychologist Steven Pinker, for example, has spoken of the 'language instinct' in that way. Linguist Noam Chomsky has said that children couldn't possibly learn language from scratch because normal human speech is full of mistakes and short on good examples to learn from.

That overlooks, however, that human language evolved as a means of sharing cognition with others in cooperative activity. The 'rules' are correlational patterns internalised from actual use in human interactions. That's what shapes its complex structure, unique productivity, and speed of transmission. After learning, very early in childhood, language helps brings culture into the mind. It is then used to vastly expand cognitive and social functions.

Shared words define objects and events as categories – chair, table, stool, and so on. By sharing the category, we can share predictabilities about what they represent – how they can be used, where to find them, and so on. Being told that an object is a table allows us to predict much more about it. But the categories also merge hierarchically into higher-level categories identified by further words ('table' is also 'furniture', also 'household goods', and so on). Such categories become extremely useful in joint thinking and action because of the further predictability they foster. They form the vast knowledge networks of the world we share, in ways not found in non-human animals.

'Verbal intelligence' is by far the most prominent aspect of intelligence testing, as described in Chapter 1. That's because the chosen verbal items are those that most reliably discriminate between social classes. Now we know why: language is not an independent set of skills or individual powers, but a culturally laden mediator between individual and culture.

Memory

To most psychologists, memory is some kind of 'store' with bigger or smaller 'capacity'. As mentioned in Chapter 1, lists of digits or nonsense syllables figure prominently in IQ tests for estimating just such capacity. From a cultural perspective, however, the idea is quite unrelated to real memory. No one has found a 'memory store' in the brain. Like all experience, memory consists of correlational patterns. And these are spread out in the millions of connections in neural networks, as described in the previous chapter. That's the case in all animals with brains and cognitive systems.

In humans, though, memory is also enshrined in cultural tools. They have evolved historically, not biologically. In preliterate societies, cultural memory included spoken and graphic forms (drawings), along with song, story, and legend. At some time in human history memories became shared in agreed marks etched on sticks and stones, or as pictograms. Even the rudimentary forms of these new tools extended social cooperation. The harvest yield, and how it's been distributed, could now be remembered for much longer periods. Memory tools became vastly more potent in later written forms, expanding the memory function, and cognitive organisation and planning. They have been augmented in more recent times by printing, libraries, calculators, and computers. In other forms those marks on sticks became the bases of numbers, developed as mathematics. Later still, that became the 'language' of science.

Science Is a Cultural Tool

It has been said that the flowering of modern science from the seventeenth century occurred when investigators started to share their work through publications and conferences. From it emerged the scientific (or what has been called the hypothetico-deductive) method. It's a highly socialised and democratic system of intense feed-forward/feedback cycles providing one of the most potent cultural tools of all. Its function is precisely to reveal predictabilities in nature beneath superficial uncertainties. That's why scientific findings often conflict with surface appearances, clashing with what seems obvious.

Those socio-cognitive tools have all become crucial to intelligence in modern societies, but we must not confuse exposure to, and assimilation of, any specific cultural tools as evidence of more or less *capacity* to acquire them. Driving on the roads is a cognitively highly demanding task, and it used to be thought that few (especially women) could acquire such complex skills. Now we are a little more optimistic!

A Brain for Culture

Modern societies comprise myriad different social roles and classes. In them, different cultural tools become assimilated by different people to different degrees. The assimilation becomes reflected not only in differences in cognition, but also in differences in the neural networks in the brain that support them. Some of these were mentioned in Chapter 6: taxi drivers, violinists, jugglers, and so on all show a cerebral 'imprint' of their activities, even in the fuzzy pictures from MRI scans. More abstract cultural differences – of values and worldviews, or tending to be individualistic or collectivist in outlook – are also reflected in differences in brain networks.

It is for engagement with such tools that our huge brains evolved. As Mervin Donald put it in *Evolution of the Modern Mind*: 'Our genes may be identical to those of a chimp or gorilla, but our cognitive architecture is not ... humans are utterly different ... We act in cognitive collectivities, in symbiosis with external memory systems. As we develop we reconfigure our cognitive architectures in nontrivial ways.'

It all amounts to a new 'method' for dealing with the world: a new intelligent system. Humans don't have the genetic and epigenetic resources to develop wings for flying, but humans fly better than any bird thanks to our deeper understanding of physical forces (thanks, in turn, to the cultural processes of science). We can move underwater better than fish and over ground faster than any other animals. And thanks to technologies like X-ray, MRI, ultrasound, infrared cameras, and so on, we can see, hear, and touch far beyond the limits of our senses.

All of that is due to the powers of pattern abstraction that have evolved to form intelligent systems. So acutely sensitive have they become in humans, in fact, that they have turned us into pattern junkies. We look for them – even simple correlations – in all that we see, hear, and do. We even create and celebrate such patterns in music, dance, games, art, and myriad creative forms. Most of all, the processes give us our individuality and personal consciousness. We only 'individuate' and become creative individuals through the psychological tools gained from cooperation in a culture. All that is part of the intelligent system that makes us human.

8 Individual Differences

Intelligent systems have been a most crucial part of evolution. They furnished adaptability in complex, changing environments. As evolved in humans, our socio-cultural intelligence fostered the construction of shared worlds far beyond the inputs of our individual senses. That has allowed us to adapt the world to ourselves, rather than vice versa, as in all other species.

Unfortunately, many psychologists, and behaviour geneticists, treat intelligence as if that course of evolution had never happened. Saddled with the agricultural model, they continue to treat individual differences in intelligence as if they were rump size in beef cattle or running speed in greyhounds. They portray the (contrived) 'normal' distribution of IQ scores as proof. And then claim it reflects a natural genetic order.

I hope you can now see why that treatment is, perhaps, one of the saddest parodies of living systems in scientific history. It really is time that we treated human intelligence, and individual differences in it, in a wider and deeper perspective. That's what I try to do in this chapter.

Order and Control

The parody has, of course, served a crucial ideological function. It has legitimised social inequalities within and between societies, making a *status quo* seem inevitable and just. As neuroscientist Steven Rose and evolutionary geneticist Richard Lewontin put it in a powerful essay in 1984, many devices for maintaining social order have been used in the past, but none has been as effective as using the apparatus of science to convince people of the levels of their own mental ability.

The device has shaped our institutions and our societies and, in many ways, the whole human world we now live in. Through its fatalism about intelligence, the class structure of our society becomes reproduced from generation to generation without too much protest. Thanks to 'our psychological advisers' (see Chapter 1) and the introduction of the 11-plus exam in Britain, the IQ test helped track hordes of us (over 90 per cent among my peers) into schools where the message was that we had no 'brains' and would only be fit for manual work. So we all started work (in my case a few days after my fifteenth birthday) officially assured that we'd found our right level and our preordained stations in life.

Today's psychological advisers, however, tend to be a little more subtle in how they present the message. In the light of the tragic history of genetic determinism, a new, and disarming, reasonableness tends to be adopted. By admitting 'environmental effects' and 'interactions', the trend has been to deny charges of genetic determinism. In this chapter I want to illustrate how the traditional message of

genetic differences ➜ brain differences ➜ intelligence differences

has been sustained anyway. To get the picture, let's consider a few recent examples.

Robert Plomin's Genie

Plomin is described as a leading behaviour geneticist of intelligence. Most of his career has been spent trying to show the importance of genes in determining individual differences. It has relied mostly on twin and adoption studies. As he admits, though, those results have always been debatable. So Plomin was quickly into the DNA (gene) sequencing enterprise, as described in Chapter 2. His 2018 book, *Blueprint*, is a culmination of that work.

Plomin is keen to emphasise the positives about finding genes for IQ, assuring the public of the good things to flow from it. For example, 'good can come from parents getting a genetic glimpse of their children's individuality – their strengths and weaknesses'. Indeed, he picks up the suggestion of others that it is the duty of parents to arm themselves with their child's genetic blueprint.

And he dangles the prospect of 'personalised education'. He does not (and cannot) say how exactly that would work. But he goes on to argue that, for employment selection, polygenic scores will be fairer than other tests because 'you can't fake or train your DNA'. A generally warm and reassuring picture is presented.

Behind those tones, however, is a no-holds-barred promotion of the old 'genes for intelligence story' littered with hyperbole and rhetorical devices: 'the DNA revolution is unstoppable'; 'the genome genie is out of the bottle'; and so on. Unembarrassed by debatable data quality, mentioned here in Chapter 2, Plomin presents research results *ad nauseum* as 'surprising', 'unexpected', 'stunning', 'astonishing', 'game changing', 'amazing', and so on. The subtitle of his book is *How DNA Makes Us What We Are*. But there is nothing in it about the 'how'.

Charles Murray's *Human Diversity*

Charles Murray was one of the two authors, the other being Richard Herrnstein, of *The Bell Curve* (1994). It acquired a great deal of notoriety for its direct conclusions, particularly about social class and 'race'. The book issued dire warnings about society's failure to ignore the results of IQ testing, presenting the stereotypes of groups at either end of the IQ ladder: one group effortlessly floats to the top of the pile, while those at the other end of the ladder go steadily downhill, 'creating fear and resentment in the rest of society'. All that on the basis of the IQ test.

In his new 2020 book, *Human Diversity*, Murray adopts an altogether more amenable, disarming approach. 'Nothing we are going to learn will diminish our common humanity', he says. 'Nothing we learn will justify rank-ordering human groups from superior to inferior – the bundles of qualities that make us human are far too complicated for that. Nothing we learn will lend itself to genetic determinism. We live our lives with an abundance of unpredictability, both genetic and environmental.'

But the old message, again, dribbles out, appealing, as before, to IQ correlations, but now galvanised by the gene-sequencing research. In his summary of main propositions, it's clear where we are being taken. These include:

- 'Human populations are genetically distinctive in ways that correspond to self-identified race and ethnicity.'
- 'Evolutionary selection pressure since humans left Africa has been extensive ...'.
- 'Continental population differences in variants associated with personality, abilities, and social behavior are common.'
- 'Class structure is importantly based on differences in abilities that have a substantial genetic component.'
- 'Outside interventions are inherently constrained in the effects they can have on personality, abilities, and social behavior.'

For all the warm tones about diversity and values, Murray doesn't seem to realise how demeaning to the very essence of humanity – that is, people's intelligent systems – those messages really are, nor how damaging they can be when policy-makers are influenced by them.

Kevin Mitchell's Account

In his book *Innate*: *How the Wiring of Our Brains Shapes Who We Are*, Kevin Mitchell emphasises the 'power in accepting people the way they are', and that we should celebrate the diversity in human nature. The book is admirable in many ways. But most of it is spent telling us things like: 'the program for a complex human brain is written into our DNA'; that DNA contains 'all the information for how all these molecules and cells should be organized'; or that the genes 'code for all the things that cells need to do their various jobs'.

Mitchell says that it is random variations in genetic programmes, along with random effects, or noise, that produce individual differences in intelligence. Sensitive to possible criticism, he admits that 'it may come across as deterministic, even fatalistic, implying that intelligence is an immutable characteristic'. So the account is sprinkled with well-meant qualifications. But it still argues quite strongly that, even beyond rare conditions, innate differences in intellectual potential exist and are measured in IQ. He speaks favourably of attempts at 'finding the genes' for IQ, as in genome-wide association studies (GWAS). More worryingly, he entertains IQ as a measure of a 'general fitness factor', as in health and mortality, creating a picture of a natural biosocial ladder.

None of this can be disputed, Mitchell says, because we now have many insights into the genetic, developmental, and neural mechanisms under-lying it. The general reader may be tempted to think that this is a reasonable framework, albeit different from the one put forward in this book. But the very deep cracks in it are manifest in its contradictions. Reliance on IQ test scores that have no scientific (construct) validity is one of them. Another is his reliance on fMRI scans, scepticism about which is now widespread (see Chapter 6). He refers frequently to modern ideas like self-organised processes, interactions in development, emergent proper-ties, and so on – but then talks of 'genetic programs' being carried out by 'mindless biochemical machines'. Above all, Mitchell alludes frequently to 'interactions' in development, yet says twin and adoption studies prove the role of genetic differences in psychological differences. He doesn't seem to realise that such studies are predicated on the assumption that such interactions *don't exist* (as I described in Chapter 2). We cannot have it both ways.

Passive Variation

By smudging inevitability, and alluding to probabilities, such accounts try to disarm charges of genetic determinism. But the drift is still very much with us, even in forms claiming to be otherwise, and easier to swallow. Even, as in Mitchell's case, where there is an admirable striving to break free, the mindset remains: deterministic genes and environments adding together in the classic nature–nurture picture. As shown in Figure 8.1, individuals vary according to the luck of their genetic and environmental lots (plus some random effects thrown in).

The model continues to be the basis for twin and adoption studies, and the gene-sequencing research on IQ. I have called it the agricultural view of intelligence. Others have called it the 'horticultural' view. But it is now as clear as can be, from the kinds of research described in Chapter 3, that it is quite unrealistic. It treats people, and their differences, as if hollow and passive recipients of genetic and environmental 'effects', almost as if they had no responsive intelligent systems at all.

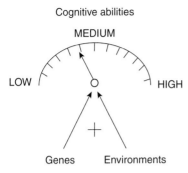

Figure 8.1   The additive (agricultural) model of individual differences.

Individual and Social

A major presupposition of the agricultural model is that intelligence is a property of a self-contained, machine-like individual. Indeed, at least since the writings of Descartes in the seventeenth century, that has been a fundamental basis of Western psychology generally. It probably explains why psychologists still struggle to reconcile individuals and their societies. Both become demeaned in the process. To understand the problem, let us return to human origins.

As described in Chapter 7, humans evolved as cooperative hunter-gatherers, probably in sporadic coalitions with other groups. There are a few remnants of hunter-gatherer groups in fringe areas of the world today: in Africa and South America, and one or two other places. They live in small self-governing bands of about 20–50 people and are nomadic, moving from place to place to follow the available game and edible vegetation. They are considered to resemble the form of humanity that existed for at least 95 per cent of our history.

The nature of individual differences among these people is interesting. As anthropologist Peter Gray explained in his 2020 article in *Psychology Today*:

> Most remarkably, unlike any other people that have been studied, hunter-gatherers appear to lack hierarchy in social organization. They

have no chief or big man, no leaders or followers. They share everything, so nobody owns more than anybody else. They make all group decisions through discussion until a consensus is reached. In fact, another name that anthropologists regularly use to refer to band hunter-gatherer societies is *egalitarian societies*. As part of their egalitarianism, they have an extraordinary degree of respect for individual autonomy. They don't tell one another what to do or offer unsolicited advice.

In another article in *Psychology Today*, psychologist Steve Taylor says:

> One of the striking things about such groups is their egalitarianism. As the anthropologist Knauft has remarked, hunter-gatherers are characterized by 'extreme political and sexual egalitarianism' … Individuals in such groups don't accumulate their own property and possessions; they have a moral obligation to share everything. They also have methods of preserving egalitarianism by ensuring that status differences don't arise.

The intelligence of individuals is clearly cultural, in the sense described in Chapter 7. Younger members follow the lead of older mentors, eventually augmenting group intelligence with experiences of their own. That means access to all deliberations and sharing of executive proceedings. Rational decisions are dispersed among the group as a whole, with fluid divisions of labour. Moreover, in an earlier blog in 2011, Peter Gray said such people 'had friends and relatives in neighboring bands and maintained peaceful relationships with neighboring bands. Warfare was unknown to most of these societies, and where it was known it was the result of interactions with warlike groups of people who were not hunter-gatherers.'

Of course, a Rousseau-esque view of the 'noble savage' may be written off by some as romantic idealism or 'primitive communism', irrelevant to today's world. Strangely enough, though, an article by anthropologist James Suzman in the *Financial Times* (1 September 2020) describes his long study of one such tribe, the Ju/'hoansi people of the north-western Kalahari, in similar terms. He says, 'the longer I stayed with them, the more I became convinced that understanding their economic approach not only offered insights into the past – it also provided clues as to how we in the industrialised world might organise ourselves in an increasingly automated future'.

Caution is needed, however, because there have been reports painting rather less peaceful pictures of such groups. On the other hand, it is known how even minimal contact with Westerners can disturb their social harmony. In a caustic review of selective accounts, anthropologist William Buckner warns, 'In reality, human beings everywhere are neither inherently freedom loving and peaceful, nor inherently coercive and violent, but can be either or both depending on their socio-ecological and cultural context.' In other words, groups and individuals can refract changing and challenging contexts in unpredictable ways, drastically influencing their perceptions, and their feelings. Let us now consider what happened with the most durable of such refractions, the consequences of which – for intelligence and much else – we experience so strongly in modern times.

Class Systems Emerged

The human socio-cultural form of intelligence became hugely successful. Populations expanded and dispersed, and small bands became wider coalitions. Sometime around 12,000 years ago wandering bands developed agriculture and became more settled. Wider trading networks emerged with the development of agrarian 'cities'. That brought more fixed divisions of labour and the first formation of social classes with unequal executive powers, rights, and privileges.

The cultural inventiveness that followed has been highly beneficial for humanity generally, not least for its technological creativity. But the division into social classes meant that cognitive connectedness to economic levers, and its key cultural tools, became confined to the few. The hierarchical ordering of populations was assisted by ideological devices, such as myths, gods, and religions. Priests and priestesses became important as mediators between gods, rulers, and people, who were advised to work well and follow the rules laid down from above.

Different classes developed their own subcultures, with different interests and beliefs, and derivative conceptions of the world and themselves. Individuals in class societies, that is, do not share awareness and engagement with key social processes equally; their intelligence will inevitably vary with their subcultures and degrees of learning in them. It is these social structures and ideologies that constitute the real environments of human intelligence. So now let us fast forward to their manifestations in modern times.

Top of the Pile

The dominant classes in modern societies comprise only around 2–5 per cent of the population. But they possess and control the key economic levers and the institutions and cultural tools that support them. Their power is often used discretely, but material wealth is a conspicuous benefit. That means all forms of stored up 'goods' produced by society as a whole but unevenly distributed among classes. It includes land and property, company shares, cars and boats, works of art, savings from income, and so on. It is passed from parents to offspring to create enormous advantages in terms of income stream, power, and privilege, irrespective of actual merit.

Big individual differences in families and their children, in different social classes, arise in that way. Wealth is used to create enriched physical environments from birth and throughout childhood: living conditions, diets, stable and predictable circumstances, and secure futures. All that ensures healthier lifestyles promoting physical growth and cognitive vitality. Inherited wealth also does much to get children well placed socially. So control of the levers is conserved across generations. Attendance at private schools (about 7 per cent of school students in Britain) is a major route to such ends. The schools are highly focused on school exams, university entrance, and futures in the major institutions.

That means networking with people in influential positions, so gaining patronage in employment opportunities, lobbying power, and mental engagement with those levers of social power. A sense of security and independence fosters booming self-confidence and sense of entitlement and place. One consequence is that we get a preponderance (over 50 per cent in the UK) of such beneficiaries of inherited wealth in powerful positions in all the institutions, especially politics. Above all else, surveys show how those in higher classes exhibit an elevated sense of control over their own situations.

The Other End

The circumstances of lower social classes are very different and have serious consequences for their children's readiness for tests and schooling. Materially, parents have constant grinding worry about money shortages, housing, and future job and social security. That depletes energy for cognition, health and vitality, and the 'extra' needed for pushing their offspring for school and long-term aspiration.

But the non-material consequences are worse. As Angela Saini says in her book *Superior*, 'Notions of superiority and inferiority impact us in deep ways.' Just feeling at the lower end of the pile – or what is called 'subjective social status' – is strongly related to test, school, and later job performance. In a paper in the journal *Self and Identity* in 2015, Benita Jackson and colleagues put this as follows: 'To internalize social status is to believe the self is responsible for it.' It all creates what researchers have called a 'double disadvantage'. Added to little material well-being is conception of personal place in the hierarchy and its explanation. One of the points of IQ testing, as well as schooling, after all, has been to get people to accept that their social position is inevitable. They thus become cognitively disarmed in relation to expectations of the major social institutions.

That view concurs with the main finding of *The Spirit Level*, by Richard Wilkinson and Kate Pickett, with analyses done in a number of countries, including the USA. The greater the inequality of the society to which a child belongs, the wider the differences in school performance. Feeling at the bottom of an even steeper social cliff has big psychological conse-quences. And those psychological effects are reflected in physiology, health, and general vigour. Wilkinson and Pickett (as reported in 2017) further analysed results from over 200 studies showing that the factors most reliably pushing up levels of stress hormones are threats to self-esteem. That is supported by a review by Robert Sapolsky in *Nature Neuroscience* in 2015: 'It is a truism that the brain influences the body and that peripheral physiology influences the brain. Never is this clearer than during stress, where the subtlest emotions or the most abstract thoughts can initiate stress responses, with consequences throughout the body [that] alter cognition, affect and behaviour.'

So, there is much evidence that perception of personal rank in the social hierarchy uniquely predicts psychological state, health, and well-being. The culture of fatalism and pessimism created by media stories about genes and IQ no doubt fosters that, too. And they are all even worse for ethnic minorities, who face the added stress of racism (see further below). Of course, in order to cope with and survive their conditions, social classes tend to have developed their distinctive cultural tools. But one thing seems fairly clear: in spite of material, psychological, and health difficulties, people in those positions are not cognitively deficient. Developmental psychologists Willem Frankenhuis and Carolina de Weerth showed that children from stressed backgrounds actually exhibit *improved* detection, learning, and memory of factors (e.g. threats and dangers) relevant to their circumstances, compared with safely nurtured peers. They are simply intelligent in other ways.

These are the real environments in which individual differences arise. Between these vast social inequalities, and associated ideologies, a deep socio-psychodrama is played in which people and their children are responsive individuals, not passive capsules. It has been all too easy to spin those individual differences as if they were inherent properties of individuals rather than the societies in which they live. Ironically, that agricultural model has not only inspired dubious genetic research, it has also led to misconceptions about the environment.

The Missing Environment

There have been decades of research into 'environmental' sources of individual differences in intelligence. Although well-meaning, it does reveal much about the underlying notions of the environment. The methods have generally consisted of questionnaires to parents, and observations and interviews by researchers visiting homes and schools. Broad factors such as parental teaching style, discipline style, numbers of toys and books in the home, family income, and neighbourhood and housing characteristics have all been recorded and graded. Correlations with IQ tests and school attainments have then been estimated.

A UK Department for Education project reported by educator Pam Sammons and colleagues in 2014 presented a fairly typical pattern. The home environment measure was based on the frequency of specific activities involving the child as reported by parents. These included teaching the alphabet, playing with letters and numbers, library visits, reading to the child, teaching songs or nursery rhymes, and so on. They were all statistically associated with later school attainments, especially when combined with other factors such as parents' education, income, quality of neighbourhood, and so on.

Such studies include pioneering efforts in difficult circumstances. And sometimes insights are gained. For example, one group claimed that pre-schoolers exposed to 'spatial' terms like *underneath* or *behind* (more frequent in middle-class homes) show better learning of mathematics in school. Others have shown how such learning is related to 'home numeracy' – the extent to which parents use numerical skills – more than anything else (including the children's IQ scores). But the studies do not get to the root of the matter. The variables are probably best viewed as *correlates* of the real bases of differences in school attainments rather than causes. That probably explains why, when such factors have been used to guide intervention programmes for young children – for example, by coaching parents or providing compensatory reading lessons – the effects tend to be small or don't last (see further in Chapter 9).

Little wonder, then, that the going model of environment cannot explain why even children in the same family are so different from one another. A 2011 commentary by Eric Turkheimer in the *International Journal of Epidemiology* is still valid: 'attempts to [identify] systematic environmental causes that produce systematic differences in outcome almost always end in disappointment'. Researchers of the environment are clearly barking up the wrong tree.

This is not to deny that many specific and severe 'environmental factors' can affect cognitive development by impairing the underlying system itself – the robust ability to interact and adapt, as the vast majority of children do. For example, there is research evidence that maternal nutrition or stress can effect brain development, and later stress sensitivity, in the child. A wide range of toxic substances, such as atmospheric lead, traffic fumes, other pollutants, and drugs, have been studied in that respect. A clearer example is the research with children who spent early childhood in the Romanian orphanages of the oppressive Ceausescu era. Having been exposed to severe material and mental deprivations, they were subsequently adopted by UK families. The researchers observed distinct consequences in reduced brain volume and surface, correlating with duration of deprivation.

For the vast majority, however, the causes of individual differences have arisen from environments at a quite different level. Adherence to the agricultural model has diverted attention from the real environment of intelligence. It has treated people as passive statistical units, subject to independent genes-plus-environment forces, and creates many problems of interpretation, as Plomin, Murray, and others illustrate. The model of passive subjects cannot explain why even children in the same family are so different from one another. So those authors have been obliged to invent another phantom 'factor'. This is the idea that the environment is really 'genetic': that it's really the children's genes making them behave in ways, and creating environments, that make them so unalike. Or it's the parent's genes that create more or less good environments for their children.

That is reminiscent of geneticist Thomas H. Morgan's warning in 1917 about 'the greatest danger of the factorial [i.e. statistical] procedure. If, for example, whenever one fails to account for a result he introduces another factor to take care of what he cannot explain he is not proving anything except that he is ingenious or only naïve.'

Genius

A major part of the mythology surrounding the idea of innate intelligence is that high achievers have their high intelligence to thank. And that's due, in turn, to their better genes. A kind of aura is created around them, deeming them to be 'gifted' or 'geniuses'. As a society, we seem to love that picture. Perhaps it excuses our personal mediocrity; that it's not our fault, so we can be happy just muddling along. Perhaps it gives us a sense of security – that in our mundane midst are the really 'bright' ones who will see us through, take us forward. Cheer them on.

It is that picture, too, that has driven the gene hunters. If there are genes for IQ they should surely be found in abundance among the gifted. So various groups have scanned DNA in blood samples from the one in a thousand individuals with the highest IQ scores. They haven't found them. Yet, in articles with titles like 'Super-intelligent humans are coming', physicist and entrepreneur Stephen Hsu has told us that soon-to-be-available genetic engineering techniques will produce super-intelligent individuals. Others have suggested that DNA scans could one day help parents select embryos with genetic predispositions for high intelligence.

Just as strangely, though, there is little objective evidence to support that picture. A number of studies have followed high-IQ children over years or decades to see if their promise is realised. First among these was Lewis Terman, designer of the most popular IQ test. He identified individuals of IQ 130+, and called his study *Genetic Studies of Genius*. Another is the study *Exceptionally Gifted*, also in the USA. The latest is the *Study of Mathematically Precocious Youth* (SMPY), which includes IQ test scores. Since it was started in the 1970s by psychologist David Lubinski, it has included several spin-off studies.

Sure enough, in all studies, the chosen few, as a group, have tended to achieve more than their low-IQ peers who are left behind. Actually, differences between the groups are not very big. What is more surprising, though, is how easily the results of such studies have been accepted. They are seized upon, for example, in support of early educational selection. But they are not well-controlled scientific studies; rather, they are more like systematic anecdotes. They involve no randomisation of conditions with control groups. Most participants have been reared in exceptionally favourable circumstances in career-focused families. Parents were well-educated members of the middle and upper classes, no doubt steeped in the right cultural tools such as numeracy skills. Most children were also either the oldest or only child in their families.

In spite of that, a major review of 40 studies published in 2017 found that the studies had low statistical power, great variability across findings, and tended to suggest causation without sufficient evidence. Further analyses have revealed that 'gifted' individuals are no more successful in adulthood than if they had been randomly selected from the same socio-economic backgrounds, *regardless of their IQ scores*. The upshot is that if children's cultural advantages are maintained throughout life, so will be their achievements. As psychologists Guy Claxton and Sara Meadows put it in the *Routledge Companion to Gifted Education*, 'both the research base and practical and moral considerations should lead us to exclude ideas of innate and unchangeable degrees of "giftedness" from our educational practice as incorrect, inhuman, and counter-productive'.

Descriptions of 'giftedness' may really be demonstrating something more general about intelligence: how fast and how far development can proceed in a particular domain through engagement with relevant cognitive-cultural interactions. After all, nearly all children acquire their highly complex native language with great speed at a very early age. And studies of giftedness do not actually explain the extraordinary creativity of thought or invention that is undoubtedly seen at times. Consider, for example, the 'heights' of achievement in scientific discovery where those who have been especially creative will usually acknowledge the role of context. Albert Einstein himself always implied how the previous theories of Maxwell and Lorentz led inevitably to the theory of relativity. He insisted that the work of the individual is so bound up with that of scientific contemporaries that it appears almost as an impersonal product of the generation.

Yet Einstein's breakthrough is still considered to be the work of a lone genius. It ignores the fact that he received a great deal of help from friends and colleagues. Hungarian-American psychologist Mihaly Csikszentmihalyi explains this in his book, *The Systems Model of Creativity*. He says, 'The location of genius is not in any particular individual's mind, but in a virtual space, or system, where an individual interacts with a cultural domain and with a social field.'

In sum, ideas do not suddenly appear like thunderbolts in individuals' heads. Rather, they incubate in the interactive spaces between individual cognitions and those shared in social culture. Through such means, individuals will always vary in many more ways than can be summarised in a single scale. They will always be more developed in some ways than others. Many are restricted by ideological and social forces, such as being stuck at a certain occupational level or social role through lack of opportunity or self-belief. But that should not be taken to predict how individuals *could* develop in different circumstances.

'Race' and Racism

Numbers of books in the home, parenting styles, and so on are not the primary 'environmental' causes of differences in human intelligence. They are merely symptoms. That is why attempts to 'compensate' for such deprivations fail (see Chapter 9). And why psychologists have failed to identify the 'missing' environment. Rather, individual differences in human intelligence emerge from the socio-psychodynamics of political landscapes (apart, that is, from a relatively few genetic mutations or extreme environments, affecting a minority of people). Problems attributed to individuals of a particular class are those of the class system, not their superficial environments or their genes.

In a sense, it seems strange to have to say this. Aristotle in Ancient Greece fully recognised that humans are 'political animals' – that we only become intelligent in participation in the politics of a society. More recently, the argument has been reiterated by philosopher-psychologists like John Dewey and others. Unfortunately, the point has been obscured by the clouds of scientific ideology surrounding the subject. As a paper in the journal *Nature* by Angela Saini put it in March 2020, 'In failing to recognize that science can be political, the scientific community allows the resurrection of dangerous ideas.'

Dangerous ideas have been very much among the accompaniments of intelligence theory. Clothing them in scientific authority has ensured acceptance by a gullible public, even when it invites a fatalism about their own possibilities in life. Among the most dangerous is the use of superficial 'signs' and stereotypes with which to prejudge the intelligence of different groups of people. Lower social classes suffer much in that way: from their own self-concepts; from impressions and expectations formed by teachers and employers; and from effects on general health and vitality. Women generally must still struggle to overcome prejudices, and sometimes scientific dogma, about their mental abilities. All '-isms' become institutionalised as the silent assumptions and conventions that govern perceptions and treatments of others, and even our science. That is nowhere more roughly felt than in the effects of scientific racism, especially that fuelled by judgements of people's intelligence.

Racism is the idea that some groups of humans are genetically – that is, immutably – inferior. Historically, racism has arisen many times as a way of legitimising conquests, colonisation, and slavery. Scientific racism, though, is the use of scientific methods, concepts, journals, college facilities, and so on, to prove it. IQ testing has been at the very centre of it for over a century. Armed with IQ scores, psychologists have told us that 'data don't lie' or 'these are the facts'.

Controversies

Readers may well be aware of what has become a familiar pattern because it soon hits the mainstream media. A self-styled genuine scientist steps forward to bravely say the unsayable: there are differences in IQ between 'races' (usually white vs black people); they are genetic in origin; and policy-makers should heed the truth. It is followed by uproar, denunciations by other scientists, student demonstrations and boycotts, threats of legal action, and so on. Defendants appeal to the 'objectivity' of scientific inquiry, aca-demic freedom, our need to face the truth, and so on. Pictures are painted of a modern-day Galileo, fighting moral and scientific 'authority' – again, all based on IQ testing, sometimes of shockingly poor quality.

Among the latest examples is the article by philosopher Nathan Cofnas, published in the journal *Philosophical Psychology* in December 2019. It called for psychologists to take more seriously genetics-based approaches to research on 'race' and intelligence. It was followed by protests from a range of scholars and the subsequent resignation of the journal's editor. More instructive is the paper by psychologist Cory J. Clark and colleagues, pub-lished in the journal *Psychological Science* in 2020. The article is about economic production of nations in relation to IQ. It concludes, among other things, that several African, South Asian, and Central American coun-tries have an average IQ below 50 (i.e. intellectually disabled, according to standard diagnostic criteria).

The dataset used by Clark and colleagues is largely that of psychologist Richard Lynn and political scientist Tatu Vanhanen, as presented in the book *IQ and the Wealth of Nations*. Those authors claimed to have measured the average intelligence of 185 countries in an attempt to show a relationship with GDP. In fact, the 'national IQ' in any shape or form was available for only 81 of those! For 101 countries IQ was simply estimated from 'most appropriate neighbouring countries' – that is, the 'known IQs' [sic] of their 'racial groups'. Even for countries tested, 'evidence' is putting it strongly: it consists of motley tests, dates, ages, unrepresentative samples, estimates, and corrections. Estimates of national IQ include tests of 108 9–15-year-olds in Barbados; of 50 13–16-year-olds in Colombia; of 104 5–17-year-olds in Ecuador; of 129 6–12-year-olds in Egypt; of 48 10–14-year-olds in Equatorial Guinea; and so on, all taken as measures of national IQ.

I expressed my concerns about such data in a review for the journal *Heredity* in 2005. At last it looks as if its currency may finally cease. As the statement of the European Human Behaviour and Evolution Association put it in 2020,

> these data are both systematically biased against some nationalities and ethnicities, and rely on an approach to understanding intelligence which lacks universal construct validity. Any conclusions drawn from these data are both untenable, and likely to give rise to racist conclusions, even where that is not the intention of the authors. To publish using a dataset which has been constructed in a wholly flawed manner violates the principles of scientific rigour.

University departments are now disowning the authors of such dubious ideas. James Watson was the joint discoverer of the structure of DNA in the 1950s. In 2019, his base, the Cold Spring Harbor Laboratory, removed his name from its graduate school because his views on race are 'incompatible with CSHL's mission and values'. The Galton Lecture Theatre and Pearson Building in University College London have been renamed. That was partly in reaction to past connections with scientific racism, and partly to the hosting on its grounds in recent years of the *London Conference on Intelligence*. Among other things, the conference entertained the issues of 'race' and intelligence and eugenics.

But many others are still at it, with their varieties of unvalidated tests, correlations taken as causes, agricultural models, dodgy estimates of class and 'race', and scant conception of humans as conscious beings in unjust circumstances. Unfortunately, the issue doesn't stay academic. Aided and abetted by far-right political groups, each episode is accompanied by an upsurge of racism. In an analysis of their activities in 2020, Aaron Panofsky and colleagues reveal 'the loosely organized, mostly-online movement of amateur science enthusiasts (with a few ties to professional scientists) aiming to corral contemporary genetics toward racial realism and hierarchy'. Intelligence, defined as IQ, is a major prop.

There are also physical attacks on streets, harassment and bullying in schools, and prejudice and bias in the institutions. As writer Hanif Kureishi put it in a *Guardian* article, 'Racism has been the grinding backdrop to my life.' This is reiterated in Angela Saini's disturbing account of a girl of Indian descent growing up in London. There have been many other accounts of how the burden of racism adds to that of the working class in general, especially in effects on self-concept and readiness for testing and schooling. Merely informing black test-takers, for example, that a test is for research and not for ability can boost performance by 10 per cent or more. Its effects on health and well-being were demonstrated starkly in the 2020 COVID-19 pandemic. It cruelly exposed the super-vulnerability to infection of black, minority ethnic, and other deprived groups.

Human 'Races' Don't Exist

I use quotation marks because it is now clear, and has been for a long time, that races, in the biological sense intended, do not exist among humans. In other species, races are groups with distinct, and important, adaptations, associated with specific habitats and with clear genetic variations to support them. What we (unfortunately) label as 'races' in humans are *social* categories, defined on superficial criteria, with all else imputed not by objective science, but presupposition.

As I explained in Chapter 7, humans, like other species, will harbour little effective genetic variation for traits that really matter, while genetic variation for those that don't matter can remain extensive. Within and between human societies there is tremendous such variation, and that's where 'racial' lines have been subjectively drawn. Hair colour? Eye colour? Round face/long face? Male pattern baldness? Deep voice versus soft voice? Across groups there are differences like that, and we can lump or split in many ways. As Angela Saini explains in her book *Superior*, 'We can draw lines across the world anyway we choose. What matters isn't where the lines are drawn, but what they mean.' In fact, the most prominent 'lumps' we choose, and categorise as ethnic groups today, reflect Britain's (and other Western countries') imperial past and colonisation.

Some authors have mischievously focused on known genetic associations with facial and other physical features, as if illustrative of cognitive functions. These include loss of skin pigment to improve vitamin D production in less sunny climates, dietary adaptations (as in lactose tolerance in European populations), or high-altitude living in the Himalayas and other mountainous regions. Others point to differences in susceptibility to some medical conditions. Similarly, clusters of some genes will distinguish almost any socially defined group of humans, purely as a result of random distribution. But it should not be surprising to anyone. Humans have always migrated; first out of Africa and then across the globe, spreading and mixing variable genes in the process. Trading relations, conquests, and colonisation have stirred the mix even more.

In recent times, 'racial' groups have tended to be defined by national or continental boundaries, sometimes assuming genetic homogeneity that does not exist. Recent DNA sequencing studies of Vikings, for example, published in *Nature* in 2020, indicates their diverse genetic origins. They came from far-flung regions of the world, not at all reflecting their blonde-haired, blue-eyed stereotype. Another indicated that the first occupants of the British Isles were almost certainly dark-skinned. Such trivia do not meaningfully represent the biology of our common intelligent system, nor the vastly greater diversity it produces.

In his entertaining *How to Argue with a Racist*, geneticist Adam Rutherford reminds us that 'there are no purebloods, only mongrels enriched by the blood of multitudes'. So a person in any one group today will have genes from just about every other major group on the planet. So-called racial differences are superficial: genetics and human evolutionary history do not support the traditional or colloquial concepts of race. Above all, there are no studies that demonstrate causal connections between differences in gene frequencies across populations and differences in intelligence.

In declaring (as could so many others) that 'racism has been the grinding backdrop to my life', Hanif Kureishi asks, 'is a different future now possible?' In the next chapter I try to provide at least some intelligent answers to that question.

9 Promoting Intelligence

The ideology surrounding intelligence has been two-fold. First, it has aimed to convince us that the social order is a consequence of immutable biology – that inequalities and injustices are natural and cannot be eliminated. Second, where problems cannot be ignored, it tells us to look for solutions at the level of the individual rather than the level of society. Undoubtedly, the story has been phenomenally successful. Nearly everyone, across the political spectrum and around the world, accepts it to some extent. A 2020 paper from the Foundation for European Progressive Studies supports that view. It reports a European survey of attitudes of the most affluent individuals to social inequalities. Although hard work and having a supportive family background are mentioned, educational aptitude and being 'academically bright' or intelligent are cited as the primary factors.

Such attitudes are reinforced by the common belief that society provides 'equal opportunities' for individuals to demonstrate their intelligence. Expensive institutions of national education have been set up with special responsibility for that. Their main function is to provide opportunities for individuals to develop and demonstrate their *learning ability*, assumed to be a measure of their innate intelligence. If they don't measure up, one way or another it's the individual's fault. That's what this chapter is mostly about.

The Intelligence in Education

Preconceptions about intelligence pervade the education system. One of the aims of education is to promote socially valued learning, of course. But its more specific aim is to sort students out according to their 'learning ability' (i.e. intelligence). The sorting is based on how much is learned of a specially arranged menu, the curriculum. Its verdicts are sometimes about 'what type' of learning the student seems inherently suited for (also referred to as aptitude). But they are also about 'how much' each seems capable of learning. Either way, their consequences for individuals' jobs and futures are enormous.

Indeed, whatever lofty aims are stated, most people see education primarily as a filtering and preparation mechanism for future employment. In the UK, how well schools are deemed to do that creates continual paroxysms of anguish among parents and children. Getting their children beyond school, into higher education and a 'good' occupation is the constant worry of parents. They scrutinise school ratings and ranks, and even move house because of them. Those who have it just invest large amounts of cash and 'go private'.

The system, its ideology, and acceptance of them, are crucial to the stable order of society, and thus to politicians who guard it. This was acutely illustrated during the 2020 COVID-19 period in the UK. No exams were conducted, so teachers' predictions had to form the main grading/selection criterion. But 40 per cent of the estimates were statistically adjusted by the Examination Boards, such as to disfavour students from less affluent areas. According to the BBC News (4 August 2020), 'The exam body says it lowered 125,000 grades that had been estimated by teachers to "maintain credibility"'. The real worry was that of promoting hordes of students beyond their supposed natural ability.

The uproar exposed the primitive notions of intelligence, and nature–nurture preconceptions on which the system is based. But that was already evident in its common metaphors. Sometimes, technical-sounding euphemisms are used, such as 'aptitude'. But terms like 'bright', 'slow', 'strong', or 'weak' are the stock in trade of the institution in describing children's learning ability. They're hardly scientific. Their crudeness was put in a nutshell by Chris Woodhead, former chief inspector of schools, in an interview with the *Guardian* on 12 May 2009: 'It's pointless trying to make children brighter than God made them', he said. Obviously equating God with DNA, he said, 'middle-class children normally have better genes', and that's why they do better at school.

The need to make the sorting seem fair, and due to nothing besides learning ability, is intense. There is genuine concern among politicians about reducing the 'attainment gap' between social classes, as well as improving the UK's lowly standing in international tables. Those goals are being pursued with ever more testing at more ages, along with school assessments and league tables. The hope is that all that assessment provides a more valid basis for prediction of future performance. But there's little to support that validity in fact. Let's take each claim in turn.

What Does IQ Predict?

Of course, IQ test scores are moderate predictors of school attainment. Test items are selected from pre-trials *so that they do just that*. Some correlation is, therefore, inevitable. But the real basis of the link – assumed to be general intelligence, or *g* – is debatable. In fact, correlations are only moderate and are highly variable across tests and across schools and populations. GCSE (General Certificate of Education) exams are the subject-based exams sat in UK schools by 16-year-olds. The average correlation between IQ and GCSE grades in the UK is around 0.5. We must also remember that a correlation may predict an outcome, but it does not identify a cause. In reviews in *Proceedings of the National Academy of Sciences*, in 2011, psychologist Angela Duckworth and colleagues point to the role of non-cognitive factors, such as motivation, as at least part of that correlation.

Factors like self-confidence also explain much of the association between IQ test and exam performance. In a large study published in the journal *Learning and Individual Differences*, psychologist Arthur Poropat found that personality factors like persistence, or 'grit', correlated more highly with school attainments than IQ. In other studies, conscientiousness – the tendency to be organised, responsible, and hardworking – is the most predictive factor across a variety of outcomes. I mentioned the role of aspiration/expectation and parental 'push' in Chapter 8. It's possible to paint all kinds of pictures from IQ correlational data, without necessarily implicating a fixed learning ability (as opposed to just learning).

School attainments are also the gateway to occupations. Through that IQ is inevitably associated, *statistically*, with occupational level, income, and status. Again, though, these are not independent measures: levels on these job-related criteria are at least partly mediated by educational attainments which are also associated with IQ, for the reasons just explained.

The question of whether IQ predicts *job performance*, however, is a different matter. Claims of moderate associations have emerged from the dubious variety of tests and statistical manoeuvres I described in Chapter 1. There are good grounds for dismissing such claims. As reported in the *British Medical Journal* in 2013, even for well-motivated medical students, IQ did not predict progress through medical school or future career. Indeed, IQ scores had only a small association (0.285) with A-level performance (A-level exams are sat by 18-year-olds in the UK). That picture was confirmed more recently with another IQ-type test, the UK Clinical Aptitude Test. One paper was titled, 'Does the UKCAT predict performance on exit from medical school? A national cohort study', and published in *BMJ Open* in 2016. Predictive correlations were weak, leading the authors to call for 'wider debates about the limitations of these measures'.

Perhaps this more circumspect picture is not surprising as exam results seem to rely far more on swotting and regurgitation than true learning ability. As Barnaby Lenon, chair of the UK's influential Independent Schools Council, said in a BBC News feature (30 March 2018): 'The best GCSE and A-level results don't go to the cleverest students – they go to those who revised in the Easter holidays.'

What Do School Attainments Predict?

If what is being assessed in schooling is 'learning ability' (rather than simply learning), a presumed stable function of individuals, we would expect predictions from it to be sustained through attainments in later education and real life. Of course, an association between GCSE and A-level performances are to be expected – they are only two years apart, and partly replicate the same learning in much the same subjects. Even so, the associations are not very high. National statistics commissioned by the Office of Qualifications and Examinations Regulation (Ofqual) in 2011 found a correlation between total GCSE points and A-level grades of around 0.5. A similar picture is presented in a report from Cambridge Assessment in 2013. The study of highly motivated medical school students, mentioned above, showed a correlation between GCSE and A-level performances of 0.56.

In 2020, the Centre for Education Policy and Equalising Opportunities (CEPEO) in London, with Oxford Brookes Business School, studied data from 238,898 pupils. The aim was to assess the extent to which GCSE performance could accurately predict their subsequent A-level results. The team found that they could only predict one in four pupils' best three A-level results correctly. Their press release says that predicting A-level grades is a 'near-impossible task'. Their paper says, 'Overall, the low rates of prediction, regardless of the approach taken, raises the question as to why predicted grades form such a crucial part of our education system.'

But the trail becomes even more murky. A-levels have become the national entry ticket to a job or university. Again, the assumption is of a quasi-objective index of individual learning *ability*. But prediction of university performance from school tests at any level is not very good. For example, a 2012 review of 13 years of research in the USA and the UK, published in the journal *Psychological Bulletin*, found that school test scores were very weak predictors of university performance. As regards UK data, it reported only a small correlation of 0.25 between A-level points and average grades at university. (Interestingly, 'performance self-efficacy' was a good predictor.)

That confirms many other similar findings. For example, a large follow-up of medical students reported in 2013 said, 'it is clear that A-levels predict medical school performance with an average correlation of 0.24'. Research published in 2018 in *Scientific Reports*, by Robert Plomin's team, reported that A-level scores are associated with only 4.4 per cent of individual differences in final degree grades (correlation 0.22). Moreover, sequenced DNA variations (the infamous polygenic scores, as described in Chapter 2) were statistically associated with only 0.7 per cent of such differences.

It is worth mentioning, finally, research published in *Nature, Science of Learning* in 2017, which looked at IQ and school test performances of adults who went to university aged 50–79 years. It found 'that age, IQ, gender, working memory, psychosocial factors, and [sequenced candidate genes] did not influence academic performance'. There's really hope for all of us, it seems!

Ironically, it is because of the poor predictability of university performance from school attainments that universities and colleges have looked to IQ-type tests for help. But a study by the UK's National Foundation for Educational Research reported in 2010 that the adoption of a reasoning test did 'not add any additional information, over and above that of GCSEs and A levels'. Meanwhile, in 2020, a number of private and state school pressure groups are looking for suitable alternative qualifications to what are deemed to be failed GCSEs.

The overall picture, then, is murky to say the least, and we may have been deluding ourselves. Does education really test an underlying learning ability, or intelligence? The report by Robert Plomin's team bears (with little sense of irony) the title 'The genetics of university success'. But the genes, along with the heavily assumed g-factor, seem to evaporate outside the self-fulfilling correlations between IQ and school performance.

And in Real Life?

What happens beyond the education system? I discussed the lack of association between IQ and job performance above. It has also been difficult to find a robust relationship between education grades and performance in work.

Much research has been done in the USA. Personnel psychologists Thomas Ng and Daniel Feldman reported correlations between degree grades and peer-rated job performance of 0.18, and with supervisor-rated job performance of 0.09. In his review in the *Encyclopedia of the Sciences of Learning* (2011), forecasting expert J. Scott Armstrong put the correlations, six or more years after graduation, as low as 0.05. He cites research from a variety of occupations that suggests that those with good college grades did no better in the job than those without.

If school or university grades were good predictors of real work competence, we would expect it to show with medical students/doctors. The study mentioned above, however, reports small and statistically insignificant correlations between A-level results and the Practical Assessment of Clinical

Examination Skills several years later. Also, correlations between A-level scores and having been promoted to the specialist registrar (or senior doctor) grade were low (below 0.2) or not statistically significant.

Even with highly selected groups of PhD students, there seems to be little correlation between their degree performance and doctoral performance. Research in the USA showed that potential supervisors cannot predict who will successfully complete a doctorate based only on students' undergraduate records. An Australian study led by health physiologist Daniel Belavy in 2020, and published in the journal *PLoS One*, replicates this concealed truth. The study found that students' performance in their undergraduate degrees had little correlation with the publications amassed during their PhDs or afterwards. Rather, these were far more linked to the congeniality of research environments they found themselves in. The situation is unlikely to be much different in the UK.

As mentioned above, some research papers point to other factors more important than an imputed level of learning ability: conscientiousness, job satisfaction, emotional intelligence, motivation, and so on. But there is also much anecdotal evidence. An article in *The Times* (5 March 2017) announced, 'When a leading financial services firm stopped using academic qualifications to select recruits it was hailed as a bold experiment to boost workforce diversity. Now it appears it may also have been good for business as a study has found that those who would not have made it under the old criteria have outperformed those who did.' The article is referring to financial services company Grant Thornton, which receives more than 10,000 job applications each year. It abandoned its requirement for a 2:1 grade for graduates, three grade Bs for A-level entry, and a B for English and maths at GCSE for its 2013 recruitment round. It subsequently found more recruits with 'poorer' degrees became high-fliers than those with good ones. Degree class was actually a *negative* indicator of future achievement.

Other companies have followed suit. In the USA, Google used to ask everyone for school exam and test scores, but don't anymore. In an interview with the *New York Times* (13 June 2013) Laszlo Bock, a vice-president of human resources, said, 'One of the things we've seen from all our data crunching is that GPAs [grade point averages] are worthless as criteria for hiring, and test scores are worthless – no correlation at all.'

On their blog in 2016, publisher Penguin Random House posted: 'On Monday 18th January we announced that we'd be removing the requirement for a degree from the recruitment process across all our jobs.' On their website the same day, group HR director Neil Morrison referred to 'no simple correlation between having a degree and ongoing performance in work and, within Penguin Random House UK, the brightest talents came from a variety of different backgrounds, not just from the top universities.'

A series of other companies have also liberalised academic requirements for applicants. For example, Ernst and Young has scrapped its former threshold for certain A-level and degree requirements and is removing all academic and education details from its application process. PricewaterhouseCoopers has also announced that it would stop using A-level grades as a threshold for selecting graduate recruits.

Learning Ability Evaporates

I may be being selective. But I think the overall picture is clear. Look at it this way. A correlation (*r*) is a measure of co-variation, as described in Chapter 1 – how two or more variables vary together. It is sometimes used to indicate how well values on one of the variables predicts those on another. It is arrived at by taking the square of the correlation coefficient; that is, multiplying the correlation by itself: $r \times r$. Accordingly, a correlation of 0.5 between IQ and GCSE scores means that IQ scores of school students will predict their attainment scores with probability 0.25 – that is, 25 per cent of the time, or one in four individuals. By the same token (as described above) IQ scores have very little predictability for final degree performance or job performance.

On the same lines, GCSE scores predict A-level scores (correlation at most of 0.6) 36 per cent of the time – or just above one-third of students. A-level scores predict degree performance at best 6 per cent of the time (correlation around 0.25). But degrees (or any other education scores) seem to have little predictability of workplace performance. In sum, from IQ to GCSE to A-levels to university to jobs, the probability of accurate prediction is roughly *zero*.

If natural ability or intelligence is the durable function of individuals that it's made out to be, then its presence seems to wane alarmingly. Instead of, say, the enduring redness of blood, it seems to be more like an already pale juice passing through a series of drastic dilutions until it's virtually washed out. Alternatively, what is really being sorted may not be intelligence at all. In which case, we seem to be more interested in desperately upholding a mythological meritocracy than fostering the true potential of young people. In the process, countless millions of lives are being laid to waste. So it's perhaps worth taking a deeper look at what is *really* being promoted.

Testing for Social Class Not Ability

Implicitly or explicitly, education is viewed as a process of 'natural selection' of innate ability. The tacit principle is that children enter the system as a more or less homogeneous beam of light into a prism, and emerge as a spectrum of social classes reflecting their natural ability. As such, schooling is seen as the ultimate 'test' of intelligence. That's why IQ tests are calibrated against school attainments, after all.

The big flaw in that reasoning, of course, is that children do not enter the system with the same degree of school readiness; opportunities equally provided, does not necessarily mean that they can be equally taken. As explained in Chapter 8, even at age five, children are boosted or shackled by prior learning, different expectations and aspirations, self-confidence, belief in their own likely abilities, and so on. I also mentioned earlier that those we label as intelligent – or bright or smart, or whatever – tend to be those culturally 'like us': as in speaking the same language, or using the same cognitive rules of engagement. They are on the same wavelength, and think in similar terms, with greater ease of engagement and self-confidence. There is much evidence that teachers are inclined to label children on such grounds from the day they enter school. And that feeds back with positive or negative effects on the child. These are all symptoms of the pre-existing social class structure. It seems highly naive to suggest that all children in school are equally free to display their learning ability on a level playing field.

Just as important, though, is the way the typical school curriculum operates – as a test of such readiness rather than, as is supposed, learning ability. In

Chapter 7 I explained how learning in humans is quite different from learning in apes or other animals. It is different in the way that shared human language is different from the stereotyped, stimulus–response signals of chimps and monkeys. Human learning takes place at a different level, in creative – not passive – interaction between individuals and their native cultures. It includes feelings and emotional, as well as cognitive, engagement. In congenial contexts, highly complex learning, as in language and social conventions, occurs quickly and effortlessly in nearly all humans.

The typical school curriculum is most unlike such socially meaningful contexts for intelligent learning. Children are rarely required to learn the forces governing the day-to-day lives of their parents and communities; how their local and national economies work; the management and distribution of resources; local and national political administrations; the structure and functions of institutions; and so on.

As early as the 1970s, psychologist Jerome Bruner was complaining about the prominence, in schools, of artificial 'made-up' subjects. They are detached from young people's social worlds, and render most school learning tedious and irrelevant. Rather, such curricula seem to be set up specifically to test children's perseverance and confidence, which, in turn, is a reflection of parental 'push', and social class background. In his best-selling work, *Dumbing Us Down: The Hidden Curriculum of Schooling*, former school teacher John Gatto shows how even reading and writing are made more difficult than they should be.

Notorious is the case of maths. In an episode of BBC's *The Educators* (24 September 2014), Stanford University professor Jo Boaler spoke of the widespread belief in the existence of a 'maths brain'. The idea that some people are simply good or bad at mathematics is ruining pupils' chances of success in the subject, she said. Having researched the way maths is taught in schools in the UK and in the USA, Boaler says pupils are too often made to think that maths is a long list of rules and procedures to be learned by rote, instead of patterns and relations from concrete experience put to socially meaningful ends. In some ways the standard curriculum is like trying to learn to swim without water, or learning to dance without music.

Over the last two decades the problem has been getting worse because of the emphasis on standardisation and testing in an essentially factory education system. 'Teaching to tests' has become a familiar complaint. Rote, remember and regurgitate, seem increasingly to be the means and measure of success, for schools and students. Ordinarily we would expect knowledge through education to be a cumulative process. That is, we would expect learning itself to increase learning *ability*. Acquiring mathematical or writing skills, for example, should accelerate learning in other domains. On the contrary, as educator Alfie Kohn warns in *The Case Against Grades*, a 'grading orientation' has replaced a 'learning orientation'. It encourages students to opt for the easiest route to grades and focus on whether it's 'going to be on the test'. That reduces the quality of students' thinking as well as depth of learning. Little wonder that achievement in schools shows little relationship with subsequent performance in university and/or in the real world.

There have been brave attempts to liven-up curricula with more emphasis on dialogue, student-centred problem-solving, learning to think, cooperative learning, and so on. In a March 2020 article in *Psychological Review*, psychologist Garriy Shteynberg and his colleagues note that learning *from* others has been a cornerstone of learning theory in education. 'In contrast', they say, 'collective learning, or learning *with* others, has been underappreciated in terms of its importance to human cognition, cohesion, and culture'. They note how problem-solving in human groups boosts collective attention, communication, remembering, and other cognitive functions. In schools, however, the 'sorting' function of the system still requires the lone learner to be pitted against a strange curriculum.

What Alternatives?

In some desperation, ministers and school managers look to the international (PISA) league tables and wonder what they are doing wrong. Some point to the high-pressure methods at one extreme. In the UK, the schools minister announced (August 2015) an extension of the 'Chinese method of maths learning', which involves highly disciplined practice with detailed arithmetical processes (e.g. solving an equation) that pupils are expected to repeat mechanically. But it is largely devoid of meaningful content or social relevance, while incurring high degrees of student stress. Others point to the other extreme, as exemplified by the 'Finnish model': a single, end-of-school exam, no standardised assessments, no sorting or streaming by ability groups, no rankings or comparisons between schools and regions. It has very high international ratings and the lowest gaps in performances between pupils.

Not that those international rankings concern the Finns too much. 'We prepare children to learn how to learn, not how to take a test', says Pasi Sahlberg, a professor of education policy, also in Finland's Education Ministry. Although acknowledging a useful side of international comparisons, he says, 'We are not much interested in PISA. It's not what we are about.' Others increasingly emphasise that workplace preparation should be a by-product of both school and university education, not its central purpose.

Promoting learning and intelligence in schools will probably need curricula that are more carefully aligned with meaningful cultural activity. Rather than rote memorising 'dead' subjects, schools need to find ways of engaging thought, knowledge research, and practical solutions to real and familiar social issues. A local shop may have a delivery logistics problem; the Town Council a records and reporting problem; the engineer a component design problem; a local band a (musical) acoustics problem; the steelworks a physics problem; a trades union a health and safety issue; the health centre a health education problem; the shirt factory another kind of design problem; the farmer all kinds of botanical and zoological problems; and so on.

Indeed, in December 2020, the *Times Higher Education* reports how some university scholars adapted the content and topics of curricula to teach students about COVID-19 in real time. It involved integrating themes on statistics, epidemics, management, and psychology. Academics reported how the courses became educational in both the practical and academic senses, as well as helping students to psychologically process the crisis. That approach should work in schools, too.

At a wider level, there are really important issues of how the economy works, issues of employment, inequalities, resource distributions, finance systems, import–export systems, foreign relations, and global economics that could be taken on board. Using such genuine issues, all the aims and objectives of any accepted curriculum could be worked through: literacy and numeracy, literature and scientific research, computer-use, local and national history, geography, physics, biology, design, commerce, and so on. But they would be worked out in meaningful contexts, apprenticing students into the logic of empirical research and critical thinking through direct experience. That would help develop abstract concepts in a grounded way. It would also engender economic sense, a sense of worthwhileness about activities in schools, as well as civic identity and responsibility.

Some educators have long been aware of the need for new approaches. In an article in *Frontiers in Psychology* in 2020, Deniz Gökçe Erbil says, 'Active learning is defined as any teaching method that engages the student into learning process. For example, cooperative learning, problem-based learning, and project-based learning are accepted as active learning methods and have been implemented for a long time.' Papers from the OECD in 2019 and 2020 argue that work-placement learning should be a mandatory element of school-based vocational educational training. But the real solution would involve turning the education system inside out to become a true font of intelligence in our young instead of suppressing it to reproduce the social class structure of society.

Compensatory Programmes

These are not arcane, theoretical issues. Politicians and educators panic over growing social inequalities. They fear that widening achievement gaps and stalled social mobility might stir social unrest. Even more pressure is being put on education as the expected panacea. At the top, more advantaged families use their economic, cultural, and social advantages to ensure their children's success. At the other end are attempts to compensate for what is 'missing' in the environments of children from less advantaged backgrounds.

Some of these have been inspired by studies with animals in 'enriched' environments – for example, bigger cages with more toys, opportunities for exercise, and social interaction. These appeared to improve aspects of brain size, richness of connectivity, and so on, as well as 'cognitive' ability (as in laboratory learning and memory tests). Enriched treatments have also, it has been claimed, reversed the damaging effects of earlier deprived environments.

In humans such treatments have been piecemeal, but further reveal the shallow view of the environment of human development described in Chapter 8. Increased 'stimulation' from toys, pictures, colourful bedrooms, and so on have been recommended. More structured games and videos have also been tried. There were claims that listening to Mozart or other classical music can make children more intelligent. But they have been largely discredited by follow-up studies.

On the other hand have been attempts, on both sides of the Atlantic, to boost intelligence and educational achievement by wider 'compensatory' interventions. Probably most famous are the Head Start programmes implemented in the USA from 1965. The aim was to prepare poor and underprivileged children for kindergarten and school. That meant involving parents in social, educational, health, and nutritional support. Some early gains in IQ scores or educational attainments were reported, but these appeared to largely 'wash out' after the programmes ceased. However, those continuing to help parents to help their children with enrichment in the form of books and specialised games and play materials have claimed more durable benefits. So the debate continues.

A parallel in the UK was the Sure Start programme that began in 1998 and continued until 2012 under politically challenging circumstances. Their basic aim was to seek ways of intervening early in childhood. Approaches were rather nebulous and evolved over time. As described by professor of human development Edward Melhuish and colleagues, all were expected to provide: (1) outreach and home visiting; (2) support for families and parents; (3) support for good-quality play, learning, and childcare experiences for children; (4) primary and community healthcare and advice about child health and development and family health; and (5) support for people with special needs, but without specific guidance as to how.

At age seven, beneficial effects were identified for 4 out of 15 outcomes, chiefly to do with parental well-being and improved 'learning environment' and disciplinary style in the home. There were no consistent differences on any of the four child educational development outcomes, or 'proxy measures of child cognitive performance'. In their review in 2018, Melhuish and colleagues are candid about the modest and variable outcomes.

The perceived failures of those efforts have convinced some educators, as well as government ministers, that the problem really lies in the individuals. That usually means in their genes. In the 1970s, IQ psychologist Arthur Jensen famously suggested that it proves the genetic bases of ability, especially between black and white people in the USA. That view still attracts much support.

More recently the blame has been placed on individual brains, suggesting the need, among educators, for 'neuroeducation'. As claimed by neuroscientist Mohamed Seghier and his colleagues, some understanding of neuroscience 'is critical when educators are looking for novel alternative intervention methods for students struggling to learn'. Appealing to MRI research, they suggest the field will move to 'both behavioral therapies and non-invasive brain stimulation' as 'targeted individualized intervention strategies'. I described the perils of drawing inferences from fMRI scans in Chapter 6. Others have protested about the shallow theory behind such proposals, and argue that neuroscience is unlikely to improve teaching in the future.

Cognitive Enhancement

Way out, often commercialised, and invoking debatable 'scientific' evidence are various nutritional supplements, pills, mild transcranial (brain) electrical stimulation, and so on. There are a number of widely used drugs that are believed to improve attention, memory, and cognitive performance. Ritalin is probably the prime example. However, the evidence for long-term benefits of such aids is thin, to say the least. They may have no more durable effect than placebos, or the temporary boost of caffeine. In a *Science* journal article titled 'The unknowns of cognitive enhancement', Martha Farah laments the lack of control and scientific regulation in the area.

Nevertheless, psychologists Earl Hunt and Susanne Jaeggi stress how 'One of the most important tasks for cognitive researchers in the early 21st century will be developing methods to improve and then maintain people's cognitive skills, *i.e.*, their intelligence.' Among these they suggest the use of mental exercises, especially memory routines, by analogy with physical exercise. On the other hand, they also recognise that such 'kitchen-sink' approaches do not help us understand the mechanisms by which any improvement is achieved.

The bottom line is that these are all directed at the symptoms of the underlying problems, not at the problem itself. It relies on the agricultural/horticultural model of children, families, and intelligence. Palliative approaches will not do. As sociologist Richard Goldthorpe said in a 2016 lecture, 'What can be achieved through educational policy alone is limited – far more so than politicians find it convenient to suppose.' I return to that matter below.

Artificial Intelligence

Over the last two decades or so, researchers and educators have looked to artificial intelligence (AI) in two ways. First, to teach us more about the brain and thus how to boost its cognitive functions. The European Union's Human Brain Project, for example, has an estimated budget of €1.2 billion. Starting in 2013, its remit has been to build a computer that, by emulating the human brain, will reveal the secrets of intelligence, and (according to project leaders) reveal 'fundamental insights into what it means to be human'.

After over a decade, progress has been debatable – but it has revealed a lot about neuroscientists' flawed views of the brain and intelligence. The brain is not a computer. Imagine a disembodied brain, kept alive in a jar, without eyes, ears, or limbs, disconnected from the 'blooming, buzzing' real world, and the cultural toolbox of human society. What would its computations tell us about human intelligence?

The other hope for AI has been as a means of augmenting, or even substituting for, human intelligence. Perhaps computers will be able to think and operate on their own, with human-like abilities, and thus save us the trouble? In a *Frontiers* blog in 2017, Duke University's Mikhail Lebedev said, 'By 2030, augmentation of intelligence with brain implants will no longer be only the subject of research.'

To be sure, many innovations, including predictive texting and face, voice, and speech recognition, have been impressive. We see AI triumphs in many spheres of communication, industry, medicine, and so on. They have been very useful and instructive as experimental tools in artificial neural networks. Like AI systems in general, they mostly consist of layers of 'wiring' in a computer programmed with complex equations known as algorithms. They are fed data until they learn to recognise patterns in the data (a process known as deep learning).

Human intelligence, however, is based on interactions on many levels, but especially between the individual brain and the socio-cultural context of which it is part. It involves context-sensitive feed-forward/feedback loops that go beyond immediate information in creative ways. In contrast, AI systems have to be trained towards very specific tasks. They can do routine procedures and computations faster than humans. But they cannot, on their own, change the 'rules' by which they do so.

As an example, consider the efforts of Google Health to (partially) replace clinicians, or at least save them time. The team brilliantly devised deep learning techniques to help diagnose common diseases, as in heart disease, breast cancer, diabetic retinopathy, and so on. In the real world, however, they found that 'several socio-environmental factors impact model performance, nursing workflows, and the patient experience'. In other words, when decision-making and action require anticipation and prediction – the essence of real intelligence – AI systems are not in the same league as human intelligence. The cooperative learning of complex tasks from relatively few examples, and extrapolating beyond them – as in human language – has so far eluded machines. This is among the reasons why others have argued that 'general', human-type intelligence can only be realised through the historical development and emotional engagement of real human minds.

Intelligence for All

As I have argued, human intelligence arises in the dialogue between individual and culture (meaning workplaces and other social institutions). One precondition for its development seems obvious: the fullest possible participation of all individuals in those dialogues. That's how specifically human intelligence evolved in those hunter-gatherer societies of not so long ago.

Put simply, if we want more intelligent individuals we must have more intelligent societies. That must mean more democratic inclusion. If we want people to think in terms of the deeper patterns in natural and social phenomena, and in less narrow conceptual channels, we need more of what philosopher Charles Handy called 'cognitive enfranchisement'.

That was curtailed by the emergence of class-structured societies not so long ago. They entailed the appropriation of the fruits of joint activities by powerful rulers, and always needed ideologies to sustain them. Attributions of innate deficiencies of various sorts has been a common device. But nothing has been as effective as using the agencies of science, biology, and intelligence testing to convince nearly everyone (it seems) of the limited mental abilities of most people. But that's just what modern pseudo-democracy has needed.

Supposed equal opportunities provided by education systems have been part of the plan. But that, too, turns out to be bogus, as I explained above. Many others agree. The World Forum for Democracy (WDF) 2016 was on 'Democracy and equality – does education matter?' It included the question of reducing attainment gaps in education. Part of the Forum's conclusion was that 'education could do little to reduce such gaps even once reformed, as its impact is very limited on the structural inequalities'.

Unfortunately, the more the structural inequalities increase, the less cognitively enfranchised people feel. The tragedy of unrealised potential has become more acute. The question is raised: if this is democracy, is it worth having? As the WDF also notes, 'recent polling indicates the highest ever recorded levels of dissatisfaction and mistrust with democracy as a system of government. Its response to a whole series of recent challenges – economic, pandemic, and indeed environmental – have disappointed millions of people. Many are questioning the capacity, competence and even legitimacy of democratic governance to address their greatest needs.'

Uncertainty creates fear. So people have been turning to symbols of leadership, order, and national identity, as in authoritarian regimes, subordinating their own critical, intelligent thinking in the process. These questions, which bear on intelligence in a wider sense, become ever more pertinent. Solutions are needed that give people a sense of agency and control, not subordination to authority. We know enough of twentieth-century history to fear the consequences of that.

However, the world is not static, and a 'frozen' concept of intelligence may have had its day, anyway. Tiger Tyagarajan is chief executive officer of Genpact, a large company engaged in digital transformation. Writing in the online magazine *Fast Company* in December 2020 (www.fastcompany.com) , he notes that advances in digital technology are transforming the command-and-control style of business management. Instead, the need for employee engagement at all levels is democratising workplaces. Reciprocity of communication and diversity of experience is what powers creativity, he says. 'Collective intelligence outperforms the old command-and-control, top-down way of running a business', he says, and, 'It must be *the* management philosophy for the way we live and work in today's world.'

Those developments reflect a deeper irony. The class system, which – as described in Chapter 8 – has been the motor of technological development (and much else less positive), may finally be creating the technological conditions of its own dissolution. And that must mean the end of the ideologies and wider institutional cultures that have sustained it. The irony is that much of what has passed for the 'science' of intelligence is now not only suspect, but also redundant, and an impediment to future progress.

Here I have tried to present a kind of natural history of intelligence. In Chapter 3, I described how the roots of intelligence, close to the origins of life, depended on cooperation among interacting components. Terms like self-organisation, teamwork, and, indeed, democracy, have been used to capture that essential nature. Without it, life would not have originated. And it has recurred at every level of evolution from the single cell to human socio-cognition. The intelligence of individuals and groups indeed depends on genuine democracy. Without it, existence is distorted and will ultimately perish.

For a long time, a specific, and narrow, concept of intelligence has been used by states and institutions as a tool for ordering people in work and society. Some scientists have played along with that. But the opposite is now needed: the intelligence of individuals engaged, by participation, *for ordering their state*. The need has never seemed more urgent, as the long-term survival of planet and species has become a serious issue. In the long journey of intelligent systems, from the first cellular aggregates to the powerful socio-cultural system in humans, it would be even more ironic to have intelligence threatened by its very antithesis – the powerful, but one-sided, authority of a few.

Summary of the Book

The subject of intelligence has been dominated by IQ testing. The first chapter analyses that in several ways. First, I show how tests are constructed largely to match prior beliefs about its social distribution. They do not have scientific 'construct' validity (being clear about what they test). Then I show how they rely on an unrealistic mechanical model of intelligence, with differences described using simplistic metaphors like power, speed, and capacity. In describing what they really *are* measuring, I illustrate that test scores seem to be unrelated to intelligent performances in real life. There have been alternative approaches, but it has been difficult to escape from the basic assumptions underlying IQ testing.

One reason for that might be the publicity arising from twin, adoption, and now gene sequencing studies. They have convinced most people that differences in IQ are linked to 'genetic influences'. Chapter 2 describes how that research relies on unlikely assumptions about genes and environments, as well as the nature of development and intelligent functions. They are based on what I call an 'agricultural model' of intelligence that treats correlations as causes. I show how the approach is highly controversial, leaves many puzzles, and has been subject to wide criticism.

That approach assumes the gene to be a kind of autonomous decision-making agent (the 'cognitive gene', we might say). Scholars seem to have adhered to it due to lack of alternative ideas. Now we have them in abundance. Chapter 3 describes the origins of intelligence in self-organised molecular systems obeying basic physical laws. The important point is that, whereas intelligence has been conceived as a form of 'adaptation' to recurring environments, life originated in *changing* environments. By definition, circumstances changing rapidly over time, involving more and more factors, are more complex. To survive in such 'constantly novel' conditions, living things needed the ability to anticipate changes in advance, and create suitable novel responses. It happened by incorporating correlation patterns in molecular networks.

One important implication is that living intelligent systems existed long before genes existed. The genes emerged later as templates for often-needed resources. The real intelligence, or 'biological cognition', lies in the system as a whole. That's a recurring theme of the book.

Chapter 4 illustrates how such systems readily collaborated and combined to survive in progressively more complex environments. That involved both incorporation *and reconfiguration* of the originals to emerge as new intelligent systems at higher levels. Sequences of coalitions emerged into physiological, behavioural, nervous, and cognitive systems. They fostered and coordinated so much else in the course of evolution.

A crucial aspect of that was the increasing importance of development. Far from being a mere executor of 'genetic instructions', I show how development is itself an intelligent system. A staggering variety of cells, tissues, and organs develop from a single fertilised egg – all with the same genomes. This explains why the development of some traits is 'canalised', while in others it's more plastic (in some cases throughout life); and why a distinction between intelligence and instincts in behaviour is misguided. It also clarifies relations between development and evolution, and provides a better understanding of 'causes' in development and variation.

We would expect the principle of intelligent systems – the assimilation of correlation patterns – to be most concentrated in the brain. I try to show in Chapter 6 how, indeed, it is. An absolutely massive expansion of inter-cell communication, and of feed-forward/feedback loops, is seen in the most important 'association' areas. Integrated patterns transcend, feedback to, and coordinate those from individual neurons and areas. Connectivity is changed in the process (learning).

More importantly, those signalling patterns interact with each other, finding patterns within patterns. Deeper correlation patterns emerge. That is now cognition. It is conspicuously evident in visual and auditory cognition, and even in olfaction. But it is mostly present in multi-sensory interactions and the organisation of behaviour. From those dynamics emerge the basic cognitive functions: learning, memory, thinking, reasoning, and so on, present even in the tiny brains of insects and worms. We can now understand how they are aspects not of 'built-in' machines or modules, but of a deeper intelligent system.

All that emerged from former free agents such as single cells becoming intensely social. But the result was not 'free agency' at another level, as in independent organism. Chapter 7 is about how animals themselves have socialised through new levels of intelligence. The swarm intelligence of social insects is one example. Other forms exist in fish, birds, and herds of ungulates. Different complexities of intelligence evolved with them according to the conditions they lived in. Cooperative hunting is particularly demanding for such a system. There are flickers of it in monkeys and apes. But conditions of survival in changing environments turned it into a major way of life for our human ancestors.

The mental demands of social cooperation became reflected in rapid brain expansion. Patterns of action between brains were assimilated to regulate thoughts *within* them. That constituted a new intelligent system that we call human culture. I described how human culture is not merely a fortuitous effect of human joint activity, but our very means of existence. Social tools are internalised as psychological tools. Predictability of changes in the world is vastly extended while individual differences take on more variable and subtle forms. That powerful intelligent system has allowed humans to adapt the world to themselves rather than vice versa.

In Chapter 8 that perspective is brought to bear on ideas and controversies about individual differences. It is contrasted with the 'agricultural model' of genes and environments that still dominates IQ theorising. I try to show how so many problems of interpretation spring from it. The chapter then describes how the real environment – the class structure itself – creates the psychological differences attributed to dumb genes and poorly described experience. That also puts into perspective what is called 'giftedness' and exceptional achievement. Finally, it critically appraises those more notorious accompaniments of the IQ framework, namely scientific racism and eugenics.

Chapter 9 describes how the ideology of intelligence has worked largely through an 'equal opportunities' rhetoric, whereby schooling is seen as a 'test' of intelligence. The abilities so accredited turn out to be rather hollow: they have little association with long-term achievements. It seems that an utterly mythical meritocracy has been erected and maintained in at least two ways. First, the psychological effects of social inequality ensures that opportunities cannot be equally taken. Second, the standard school curriculum is more designed to test social background than genuine learning of useful knowledge. That also explains the failures of compensatory education programmes. Finally, I offer some views and recommendations on intelligence and participatory democracy.

Summary of Common Misunderstandings

Intelligence can be measured in individuals by IQ tests. That cannot be so because they are not based on a functional understanding of intelligence. Rather, scores merely quantify an individual's rank with respect to other pre-existing impressions (such as educational attainments and social class).

Intelligence can be defined in terms of a singular 'brain power' or capacity reflecting the physiological efficiency of the brain. Physiology itself cannot be reduced to such a singular index of efficiency and modern biology shows the organism is not a machine.

Performances of individuals on different IQ-type tests inter-correlate, suggesting a 'general intelligence' factor called 'g'. Correlations are not causes and, in the absence of clarity about the nature of intelligence, there are other possible (cognitive and non-cognitive) explanations for those covariations.

IQ measures ability for complex problem-solving and future performance at work. There are many examples of complex problem-solving that have little association with IQ test performance. And whether IQ predicts job performance is debatable. Rather, IQ testers seem to elevate one particular set of learned cognitive functions, related to social class background, above all others and simply assume their unique complexity.

Individual differences in intelligence can be analysed into genetic and environmental components to see which is most important. This involves an 'agricultural' model of heritability estimation. It assumes that genes can be treated as independent 'charges' that simply add up to make individuals' intelligence level. Interactions with other genes or environmental factors are not considered. Both the model, and the aims intended, are now discredited.

Correlations from twin, adoption, and DNA sequencing studies tell us how much individual differences in intelligence are caused by genetic differences (called heritability). These are all based on the (invalid) additive model just mentioned (as well as often-dubious testing). And it assumes that correlations are causes. DNA sequencing studies also have the problem of 'population stratification', whereby irrelevant genetic variants correlate with IQ through historical population movements and cultural practices (such as selective mating). Because of interactive systems, the pursuit of heritability estimates is dubious because, except for rare (controlled agricultural or disease) conditions, they will be highly variable across circumstances and populations.

Intelligence must have originated in genes at the beginnings of life, and determined the course of evolution; so genes must still determine the forms of intelligence and individual differences in it, to some extent. Forms of intelligent life – as self-organised molecular ensembles – probably existed long before genes. Genes emerged later to provide readily available resources for such intelligent systems as required. Genetic evolution has primarily followed the evolution of intelligent systems, not vice versa.

DNA genes contain 'genetic programmes' for intelligence, differences in which create individual differences in intelligence. That's not the way genes enter into biological development and function, and no such programmes have been described. Genes do not initiate any biological activities as autonomous agents. Rather, they are servants to intelligent systems at many levels, not conductors. There are no 'genes for intelligence' (see *Understanding Genes*).

It must be possible – at least theoretically – to draw a 'map' from genes to the forms and functions of intelligence and individual differences in them. Only in a minority of 'single gene' (sometimes called Mendelian) or disease traits. Otherwise, genes are used in a wide variety of ways, in alternative pathways (broadly called 'epigenetic'), according to the dynamics of the organism as a whole in a constantly changing environment.

Intelligence is a product of evolution through 'survival of the fittest' criteria. That implies being shaped to fit a narrow, and recurring, aspect of the experienced environment. Intelligent systems emerged through relations between components because they were better able to survive in *changing* environments. In fact, intelligent systems, especially in development, helped to direct subsequent evolution.

Intelligence exists in all animals and differences are a matter of degree, not kind. Indeed (and arguably in plants, too). But from the first origins, 'higher' systems emerged according to the complexity of environmental change they could survive in. That meant both incorporation *and reconfiguration* of antecedent components. So it's both: differences in degrees *and* kinds, hand in hand.

The development of all functions including intelligence is the unfolding of a plan in the genome.   It's impossible to envisage such a plan in strings of inert chemicals (DNA). Besides, a vast variety of cells, tissues, and functions all emerge from original stem cells containing the same genomes. Development is itself a self-organised, intelligent process reliant on interactions between cells and tissues and the outside environment. It is also related to evolutionary history: 'canalisation' of development is favoured in some traits; developmental plasticity in others. Some intelligent systems foster life-long plasticity, too.

Individual potential is present in the genome and realised or not according to the environment experienced.   Current ideas do not support such preformation/predetermination, either in form or in level of intelligence. It would, in any case, be dysfunctional in changing environments where more adaptable processes are needed for survival. Instead, potential is created *in the course of* development by assimilation of correlation patterns from the environment (in humans, cultural tools).

Human intelligence is just elaborate ape intelligence.   No, it's not – there was a different route to distinctly human intelligence. Apes cooperate in a perfunctory manner. But even early human species relied on cooperative hunting. That presented social environments (i.e. other individuals to coordinate with) far more complex than any physical environments. It was supported by massive brain expansion and the emergence of cultural intelligence.

Intelligence resides in the brain, a kind of advanced machine with clever built-in processing. All that we now know about the brain shows that such metaphors are misleading. The assimilation of correlation patterns is what's crucial. That's what brains do. The parts of the brain evolved for intelligent functions are dynamic learning systems in which spatio-temporal signalling is continually revising processing. Built-in processing would be a cognitive straitjacket.

Intelligence and individual differences reside in the 'wiring' of the brain. It depends on what you mean. Basic wiring of neurons and neuron groups permit some basic functions. But those functions become eclipsed by emergent activity. Millions of feed-forward/feedback circuits condense detail and boost predictability by relating current inputs to learned contexts. That involves continual reconfiguring of wiring, some aspects of which will inevitably reflect the correlation structure of individual experience. Those are qualitative differences (called experience-dependent wiring), not quantitative ones.

Human intelligence has produced human culture rather than vice versa. That is to misunderstand the nature of culture. Humans survived and evolved in extremely challenging circumstances. They did so through cooperative organisation and the social and material tools that emerged. Those tools, and their refractions through individual minds, are what constitutes human intelligence. They have co-evolved and cannot be separated.

Intelligence is a function/property of the individual. This has more to do with the ideology of Western political economics and mechanical thinking than psychology or biology. Of course, even an individual cell in a multicellular being has intelligence of what to do. But it is derivative from the intelligence of the system as a whole. Similarly at the human level: individual intelligence is derivative of the culture from which it is inseparable – albeit in an even more interactive and creative way. Broadly, people only 'individuate' in the midst of a culture.

Individual differences in intelligence are partly genetic and partly environmental. The trouble with that view is that it implies there's nothing 'in between'. There is, broadly, the organism, with intelligent systems at various (but integrated) levels. Separately and together they predict futures from current and past environmental structure, using genes in the process, but not determined by them. Except for special cases, attempts to map from genetic or environmental differences to trait differences will be futile.

We can boost human intelligence in the next and future generations through selective breeding or genetic engineering. Genes are not related to intelligence in the way presupposed here. Creative and adaptable processes of intelligent systems will always defy such attempts (except in the case of peripheral traits or those selected in agricultural production). Moreover, the simple logic may conceal hidden dangers, such as developmental anomalies.

The existence of gifted individuals or geniuses surely proves that intelligence is innate. Actually, research shows that such individuals are really gifted in highly fortuitous family backgrounds and/or working contexts. Related studies show how creative intelligence is a product of feed-forward/feedback interaction between individuals and colleagues around well-defined problems.

People from different historical backgrounds and ethnic groups have different genes, so it's possible they will have different levels of intelligence, too. That proposition is the basis of scientific racism, inviting different treatments for different groups. It seriously misunderstands the nature of human intelligence and of human genetic variation. Groups cannot be cleanly distinguished in such ways. Besides, intelligence can no more be characterised by a singular level than physiology can.

We can boost individual intelligence with suitable environmental treatments. It depends on what we mean by 'environment'. Attempts based (broadly) on an agricultural model have not been very fruitful. An intelligent systems view suggests that reduced social inequalities and greater participatory democracy might be.

With equal opportunities, education is a good 'test' of individual intelligence. That is probably a naive view. First, different social backgrounds ensure that opportunities cannot be equally taken. Second, the nature of the conventional curriculum makes schooling more a test of social background than learning ability. Research shows that test scores, either of IQ or of educational attainments, have little association with later performance in the real world.

This book suggests that we're all equal in intelligence. Surely that cannot be right? We must stop thinking about intelligence in the way we think about height and bell curves. Intelligence does not exist as a mechanical phenomenon defined by a single metric such as strength, power, or capacity. Like physiology, or the immune system, intelligence evolved as highly interactive systems, able to create adaptability for survival in changing environments. That means vast creativity and diversity of form. In humans, new forms and varieties are constantly created by cultural interaction. At any one time some people will have assimilated those forms more than other people; and (as with languages) they may have assimilated a wider *variety* of them than other people. They will have done so for a variety of historical and social reasons. Genes are used in such processes. But, except in rare conditions, gene variations do not map directly onto variations in culturally based intelligence. And that's for the best of biological reasons.

References

Chapter 1

On Herbert Spencer: *Encyclopædia Britannica*: www.britannica.com/EBchecked/topic/559249/Herbert-Spencer.

Probably the most accessible account of the history of IQ testing from Galton onwards, including Alfred Binet's work, though tending to favour IQ testing in general: Mackintosh, N. J. (2011). *IQ and Human Intelligence*. Oxford: Oxford University Press.

Johnson, R. C., McClearn, G., Yuen, S., *et al.* (1985). Galton's data a century later. *American Psychologist*, 40: 875–892.

On medieval urinalysis: *What medieval doctors used to do with urine was once disgusting, cutting edge medicine*: www.viralnova.com/urine-doctors. A fairly light introduction to Binet and his legacy: Byford, J., McAvoy, J., and Banyard, P. (2014). *Investigating Intelligence*. Milton Keynes: Open University Press.

For a history of eugenics in IQ and education: Chitty, C. (2007). *Eugenics, Race and Intelligence in Education*. London: Bloomsbury. Gould, S. J. (1996). *The Mismeasure of Man*. New York: W.W. Norton.

On test validity: Markus, K., and Borsboom, D. (2013). *Frontiers of Validity Theory: Measurement, Causation, and Meaning*. New York: Routledge.

A useful summary of the myriad tests, the results of which are used by Schmidt and colleagues: Bertua, C., Anderson, N., and Salgado, J. F. (2005). The predictive validity of cognitive ability tests: a UK meta-analysis. *Journal of Occupational and Organizational Psychology*, 78: 387–409.

On the 'Flynn effect': Flynn, J. R. (2013). *Are We Getting Smarter? Rising IQ in the Twenty-First Century*. Cambridge: Cambridge University Press.

On prior experience and complex problem solving in simulated real-world contexts: Süß, H.-M. and Kretzschmar, A. (2018). Impact of cognitive abilities and prior knowledge on complex problem solving performance: empirical results and a plea for ecologically valid microworlds. *Frontiers in Psychology*, 9: 626. DOI: 10.3389/fpsyg.2018.00626.

A fuller account of what IQ tests (really) test, including non-cognitive factors: Richardson, K. and Norgate, S. H. (2014). Does IQ measure ability for complex cognition? *Theory & Psychology*, 24: 795–812. See also Lee, J. and Stankov, L. (2017). *Noncognitive Psychological Processes and Academic Achievement*. London: Routledge.

A collection of 'many different perspectives' is presented in Sternberg, R. J. (2018). *The Nature of Human Intelligence*. Cambridge: Cambridge University Press. It includes a chapter by Howard Gardner, but broadly illustrates the continuing dominance of the IQ framework. Sternberg's website is www.robertjsternberg.com.

Chapter 2

Descriptions and critiques of Fisher's genetic model: Barton, N., Hermisson, J., and Nordborg, M. (2019). Population genetics: why structure matters. *eLife*, 8: e45380. DOI: 10.7554/eLife.45380; Nelson, R. M., Pettersson, M. E., and Carlborg, O. (2013). A century after Fisher: time for a new paradigm in quantitative genetics. *Trends in Genetics*, 29: 669–676; Portin, P. and Wilkins, A. (2017). The evolving definition of the term 'Gene'. *Genetics*, 205: 1353–1364; Fisher, R. A. (1951). Comment. *British Agricultural Bulletin*, 4: 217–218.

Earlier critique of twin studies and their wider social and scientific implications: Kamin, L. J., Rose, S., and Lewontin, R. C. (1984). *Not in Our Genes: Biology, Ideology and Human Nature*. New York: Pantheon Books.

Links to Jay Joseph's more recent critiques: www.madinamerica.com/2020/02/exploding-twin-study-myth; https://thegeneillusion.blogspot.com/2020/08/its-time-to-radically-reevaluate-reared_9.html.

Description of online testing in a large twin study: Haworth, C. M. A., Harlaar, N., Kovas, Y., *et al.* (2007). Internet cognitive testing of large samples needed in genetic research. *Twin Research and Human Genetics*, 10: 554–563.

Average IQ is higher in adopted children: Kendler, K., Turkheimer, E., Ohlsson, H., *et al.* (2015). Family environment and the malleability of cognitive ability: a Swedish national home-reared and adopted-away cosibling control study. *Proceedings of the National Academy of Sciences*, 112(15): 4612–4617.

On GWAS/PGS for education/intelligence: Lee, J. J., Wedow, R., Okbay, A., *et al.* (2018). Gene discovery and polygenic prediction from a genome-wide association study of educational attainment in 1.1 million individuals. *Nature Genetics*, 50: 1112–1121.

National Institute of Health website on SNPs: https://ghr.nlm.nih.gov/primer/gen omicresearch/snp. On the role of interactions: Morgante, F., Huang, W., Maltecca, C., and Mackay, T. F. C. (2018). Effect of genetic architecture on the prediction accuracy of quantitative traits in samples of unrelated individuals. *Heredity*, 120: 500–514.

For problems with GWAS/polygenic scores: Richardson, K. (2020). Polygenic scores are an even bigger social hazard. *Progress in Biophysics and Molecular Biology*, 153: 13–16; Mostafavi, H. *et al.* (2020). Variable prediction accuracy of polygenic scores within an ancestry group. *eLife*, 9: e48376. DOI: 10.7554/eLife.48376.

The study finding association between the polygenic score of a weed and a country's GDP: Kern, A. (2020). Creating a PGS for GDP using Arabidopsis data: https://github.com/andrewkern/gdp_pgs/blob/master/araThal.ipynb.

Chapter 3

For life origins: Steel, M., Hordijk, W., and Xavier, J. C. (2019). Autocatalytic networks in biology: structural theory and algorithms. *Journal of the Royal Society Interface*, 16(151): 20180808. DOI: 10.1098/rsif.2018.0808. Goldford, J. E. and Segrè, D. (2018). Modern views of ancient metabolic networks. *Current Opinion in Systems Biology*, 8: 117–124.

Bruce Damer's blog post: *Niche Construction*, 8 May 2019, https://extendedevo lutionarysynthesis.com/the-hot-spring-hypothesis-for-the-origin-of-life-and-the-extended-evolutionary-synthesis.

On RNA as original catalysts: Shen, L. and Ji, H.-F. (2011). Small cofactors may assist protein emergence from RNA world: clues from RNA–protein complexes. *PLoS One*, 6(7): e22494. DOI: 10.1371/journal.pone.0022494. A popular article by Zimmer, C. (2014). A tiny emissary from the ancient past, *New York Times*, 25 September, relates that role to today's viruses and 'viroids' (basically RNA viruses without their protein jackets). McGregor, S., Vasas, V., Husbands, P., and Fernando, C. (2012). Evolution of associative learning in chemical networks. *PLoS Computational Biology*, 8: e1002739. DOI: 10.1371/journal.pcbi.1002739.

On the subordinate role of natural selection in natural conditions: Pujol, B., Blanchet, S., Charmantier, A., *et al.* (2019). The missing response to selection in the wild. *Trends in Ecology and Evolution*, 33: 337–346.

On survival in changeable environments: Richardson, K. (2020). In the light of the environment: Evolution through biogrammars not programmers. *Biological Theory*, 15: 212–222.

On the subordinate role of the genes: Noble, D. (2016). *Dancing to the Tune of Life*. Cambridge: Cambridge University Press; Baverstock, K. (2021). The gene: an appraisal. *Progress in Biophysics and Molecular Biology*. DOI: 10.1016/j.pbiomolbio.2021.04.005.

Discussions of cognitive biology: Baluška, F. and Levin, M. (2016). On having no head: cognition throughout biological systems. *Frontiers in Psychology*, 7: 902. DOI: 10.3389/fpsyg.2016.00902. On similar lines: Levin, M. and Dennet, D. C. (2020). Cognition all the way down. *Aeon*: https://aeon.co/essays/how-to-understand-cells-tissues-and-organisms-as-agents-with-agendas (this has been criticized for allusions to human-like agency and purpose).

A more extended discussion on the nature of the gene in relation to development and function: Kampourakis, K. (2022). *Understanding Genes*. Cambridge: Cambridge University Press.

On mismatch between gene products and cell outcomes: Piran, M., Karbalace, R., Piran, M., *et al.* (2019). Do signaling networks and whole-transcriptome gene expression profiles orchestrate the same symphony? *bioRxiv* preprint: http://dx.doi.org/10.1101/643866; Yang, C. Farias, F. G., Ibanez, L., *et al.* (2020). Genomic and multi-tissue proteomic integration for understanding the biology of disease and other complex traits. *medRxiv* preprint: https://doi.org/10.1101/2020.06.25.20140277.

Bizzarri, M., Brash, D. E., Briscoe, J., *et al.* (2019). A call for a better understanding of causation in cell biology *Nature Reviews Molecular Cell Biology*, 20(5): 261–262.

Chapter 4

Evolution/adaptation in changing environments: Richardson, K. (2020). In the light of the environment: Evolution through biogrammars not programmers. *Biological Theory*, 15: 212–222.

On the 'complexity' problem: Duclos K. K., Hendrikse, J. L., and Jamniczky, H. A. (2019) Investigating the evolution and development of biological complexity under the framework of epigenetics. *Evolution and Development*. DOI: 10.1111/ede.12301.

On slime mould intelligence: Lee, J., and Zhang, L. (2015). The hierarchy quorum sensing network in *Pseudomonas aeruginosa*. *Protein & Cell*, 6(1): 26–41. Vallverdú, J., Castro, O., Mayne, R., *et al.* (2018). Slime mould: the fundamental mechanisms of biological cognition. *Biosystems*, 165: 57–70. And an entertaining article by Levy, M. G. (2020). A slime mold changes its mind: an interview with slime mold scientist Audrey Dussutour. *Massive Science*: https://massivesci.com/articles/slime-mold-ants-audrey-dussutour-breakthrough/?s=09. Cavalier-Smith, T. (2017). Origin of animal multicellularity: precursors, causes, consequences: the choanoflagellate/sponge transition, neurogenesis and the Cambrian explosion. *Philosophical Transactions of the Royal Society B*, 372: 20150476. Sogabe, S. Hatleberg, W. L., Kocot, K. M., *et al.* (2019). Pluripotency and the origin of animal multicellularity. *Nature*, 570: 519–525.

On anticipatory processes in physiology: Woods, S. C. and Ramsay, D. S. (2007). Homeostasis: beyond Curt Richter. *Appetite*, 49: 388–398. Ivanov, P. C. and Bartsch, R. P. (2014). Network physiology: mapping interactions between networks of physiologic networks. In D'Agostino, G. and Scala, A. (eds), *Networks of Networks: The Last Frontier of Complexity*. New York: Springer. Blanchard, D. C., McKittrick, C. R., Blanchard, R. D., and Hardy, M. P. (2002). Effects of social stress on hormones, brain and behaviour. Part I. In Pfaff, D. W., Arnold, A. P., Farbach, S. E., *et al.* (eds), *Hormones, Brain and Behaviour*. New York: Elsevier.

On mechanical (and better) theories of behaviour: Gomez-Marin, A. and Ghazanfar, A. A. (2019). The life of behavior. *Neuron*, 104. DOI: 10.1016/j.neuron.2019.09.017

On functional aspects of the nervous system of a roundworm: Pan, R. K., Chatterjee, N., and Sinha, S. (2010). Mesoscopic organization reveals the constraints governing *Caenorhabditis elegans* nervous system. *PLoS One*, 5 (2): e9240. DOI: 10.1371/journal.pone.0009240.

On primitive brains: Pagán, O. R. (2019). The brain: a concept in flux. *Philosophical Transactions of the Royal Society B*. DOI: 10.1098/rstb.2018.0383.

Chapter 5

How cells differentiate: Stathopoulos, A. and Iber, D. (2013). Studies of morphogens: keep calm and carry on. *Development*, 140: 4119–4124. Small, S. and Briscoe, J. (eds) (2020). *Gradients and Tissue Patterning*. London: Elsevier.

For feed-forward/feedback loops in stem cell differentiation: Pardo-Saganta, A., Tata, P. R., Law, B. M., *et al.* (2015). Parent stem cells can serve as niches for their daughter cells. *Nature*, 523: 597–601. Waddington, C. H. (1968–72). *Towards a Theoretical Biology* (in 4 volumes). Edinburgh: Edinburgh University Press.

Molecular biology of canalisation: Balaskas, N., Ribeiro, A., Panovska, J., *et al.* (2012). Gene regulatory logic for reading the sonic hedgehog signaling gradient in the vertebrate neural tube. *Cell*, 148: 273–284. Mringa Sur's website: www.surlab.org.

A comprehensive review of developmental plasticity: Kelly, S. A., Panhuis, T. M., and Stoehr, A. M. (2012). Phenotypic plasticity: molecular mechanisms and adaptive significance. *Comprehensive* Physiology, 2: 1417–1439.

On epigenetics of development, with special reference to brain, stress, and nutrition: Nugent, B. M. and McCarthy, M. M. (2015). Epigenetic influences on the developing brain: effects of hormones and nutrition. *Advances in Genomics and Genetics*, 5: 215–225. Silver, D. L., Rakic, P., Grove E. A., *et al.* (2019). Evolution and ontogenetic development of cortical structures. In Singer, W., Sejnowski, T. J., and Rakic, P. (eds), *The Neocortex*. Cambridge, MA: MIT Press.

A lively review of (life-long) brain plasticity: Engleman, D. (2015). *The Brain*. Edinburgh: Canongate Books. See also Lövdén, M., Wenger, E., and

Mårtensson, J. (2013). Structural brain plasticity in adult learning and development. *Neuroscience and Biobehavioral Reviews*, 37: 2296–2310.

On the distinction between instincts and intelligence: Bateson, P. (2017). *Behaviour, Development and Evolution*. London: Open Book Publishers. Blumberg, M. S. (2017). Development evolving: the origins and meanings of instinct. *WIREs Cognitive Science*, 8: e1371. DOI: 10.1002/wcs.1371.

On causes and difference-makers: DiFrisco, J. and Jaeger, J. (2020). Genetic causation in complex regulatory systems: an integrative dynamic perspective. *BioEssays*, 42: 1900226. See also Kampourakis, K. (2019). Genetics makes more sense in the light of development. In G. Fusco (ed.), *Perspectives on Evolutionary and Developmental Biology*. Padova: Padova University Press.

A modern evolutionary-developmental perspective is provided by Wallace Arthur in *Evo-Devo* in this series. See also Lickliter, R. (2017). Developmental evolution. *WIREs Cognitive Science*, 8(1–2). DOI: 10.1002/wcs.1422.

Chapter 6

The quotations from Kevin Mitchell are from his blog, Wiring the Brain (4 January 2020), a lively centre of discussion on the latest research. Global Brain Workshop 2016 Attendees (2016). Global challenges for the brain sciences. 2016 Conference Abstract. *F1000Research*, 5: 2873. Pagán, O.R. (2019). The brain: a concept in flux. *Philosophical Transactions of the Royal Society B*. DOI: 10.1098/rstb.2018.0383 Cobb, M. (2018). *The Idea of the Brain*. London: Profile Books.

On feed-forward/feedback processing in the brain: Bányai, M., Lazar, A., Klein, L., et al. (2019). Stimulus complexity shapes response correlations in primary visual cortex. *Proceedings of the National Academy of Sciences*, 116(7): 201816766. Bao, S. (2015). Perceptual learning in the developing auditory cortex. *European Journal of Neuroscience*, 41: 718–724. Schrader, S., Gewaltig, M-O., Körner, U., and Körner, E. (2009). Cortext: a columnar model of bottom-up and top-down processing in the neocortex. *Neural Networks*, 22: 1037–1200 (a special issue devoted to cortical columns).

On dynamic systems in the brain: Brakespear, M. (2017). Dynamic models of large-scale brain activity. *Nature Neuroscience*, 20: 340–352.

On olfaction: Barwich, A.-S. (2019). A critique of olfactory objects. *Frontiers in Psychology*, 10: 1337. DOI: 10.3389/fpsyg.2019.01337. Freeman, W. J. (1999). *How Brains Make Up Their Minds*. London: Weidenfeld and Nicolson.

On audition: Bao, S. (2015). Perceptual learning in the developing auditory cortex. *European Journal of Neuroscience*, 41: 718–724.

On experience-dependence in brain networks: Lövdén, M., Wenger, E., Mårtensson, J., *et al.* (2013). Structural brain plasticity in adult learning and development. *Neuroscience and Biobehavioral Reviews*, 37: 2296–2310.

On emotion and intelligence: Okon-Singer, H. Hendler, T., Pessoa, L., and Shackman, A. J. (2015). The neurobiology of emotion–cognition interactions: fundamental questions and strategies for future research. *Frontiers in Human Neuroscience*, 9: 58. DOI: 10.3389/fnhum.2015.00058.

On efforts to relate intelligence to size and other aspects of brain: Allen, J. S. (2009). *The Lives of the Brain*. Cambridge, MA: The Belknap Press.

On the effects of extreme deprivation on physical aspects of the brain: Mackes, N. K., Golm, D., Sarkar, S., *et al.* (2020). Early childhood deprivation is associated with alterations in adult brain structure despite subsequent environmental enrichment. *Proceedings of the National Academy of Sciences USA*, 117: 641–649. Nugent, B. M. and McCarthy, M. M. (2015). Epigenetic influences on the developing brain: effects of hormones and nutrition. *Advances in Genomics and Genetics*, 5: 215–225.

On the unreliability of MRI scans: Botvinik-Nezer, R. Holzmeister, F., Camerer, C. F., *et al.* (2020). Variability in the analysis of a single neuroimaging dataset by many teams. *Nature*, 582: 84–88. Weinberger, D. R. and Radulescu, E. (2020). Structural magnetic resonance imaging all over again. *JAMA Psychiatry*. DOI: 10.1001/jamapsychiatry.2020.1941.

On the notion of fixed wring: Salehi, M., Greene, A. S., Karbasi, A., *et al.* (2020). There is no single functional atlas even for a single individual: functional parcel definitions change with task. *NeuroImage* 208: 116366.

Chapter 7

On the problems of a competitive-selectionist view of intelligence: Smith, S. E. (2020). Is evolutionary psychology possible? *Biological Theory*, 15: 39–49.

For social hunting and brain size: Drea, C. M. and Carter, A. N. (2009). Cooperative problem solving in a social carnivore. *Animal Behaviour*, 78: 967–977. Holekamp, K. E. and Benson-Amram, S. (2017). The evolution of intelligence in mammalian carnivores. *Interface Focus*. DOI: 10.1098/rsfs.2016.0108.

On the 'social brain' idea: Dunbar, R., Gamble, C., and Gowlett, J. (2017). *Thinking Big: How the Evolution of Social Life Shaped the Human Mind*. New York: Thames and Hudson.

Considering brain size in relation to wider ecological demands in primates: Charvet, C. J. and Finlay, B. L. (2012). Embracing covariation in brain evolution: large brains, extended development, and flexible primate social systems. In Homan, M. A. and Falk, D. (eds), *Progress in Brain Research*. Amsterdam: Elsevier.

On cooperative hunting in chimpanzees: Boesch, C., Boesch, H., and Vigilant, L. (2006). Cooperative hunting in chimpanzees: kinship or mutualism? In Kappeler, P.M. and van Schaik, C. P. (eds), *Cooperation in Primates and Humans*. Berlin: Springer.

For the conventional primate-centred view of culture (or 'cultural primatology'): Humle, T. and Newton-Fisher, N. E. (2013). Culture in non-human primates: definitions and evidence. In Ellen, R. F., Lycett, S. J. and Johns, S. E. (eds), *Understanding Cultural Transmission in Anthropology: A Critical Synthesis*. New York: Berghahn Books.

For an outline of human evolution: Stringer, C. and Galway-Witham, J. (2017). Palaeoanthropology: on the origin of our species. *Nature*, 546: 212–214; Antón, S. C., Potts, R., and Aiello, L. C. (2014). Evolution of early *Homo*: an integrated biological perspective. *Science*, 345. DOI: 10.1126/science.12368280. Gabora, L. and Russon, A. (2011). The evolution of human intelligence. In Sternberg, R. and Kaufman, S. (eds), *The Cambridge Handbook of Intelligence*. Cambridge: Cambridge University Press.

On wide resource networks of stone-age humans: Tollefson, J. (2018). Advances in human behaviour came surprisingly early in Stone Age. *Nature*, 555: 424–425.

For another view on the importance of cooperation: Corning P. (2018). *Synergistic Selection: How Cooperation Has Shaped Evolution and the Rise of Humankind*. Singapore: World Scientific.

On the variety of approaches to 'collective intelligence': Nguyen, N. T., Kowalczyk, R., Mercik, J., and Motylska-Kuźma, A. (eds) (2020). *Transactions on Computational Collective Intelligence XXXV*. New York: Springer. Woolley, A. W., Aggarwal, I., and Malone, T. W. (2015). Collective intelligence and group performance. *Current Directions in Psychological Science*, 24(6): 420–424. See also papers from the MIT Center for Collective Intelligence.

For the theory of cultural tools: Bruner, J. S. (1985). Vygotsky: a historical and conceptual perspective. In J. V. Wertsch (ed.), *Culture, Communication and Cognition: Vygotskian Perspectives*. Cambridge: Cambridge University Press. Vygotsky, L. S. (1988). The genesis of higher mental functions. In Richardson, K. and Sheldon, S. (eds), *Cognitive Development to Adolescence*. Hove: Erlbaum.

Intersubjectivity in development: Beebe, B. and Bahrick, L. E. (2016). A systems view of mother–infant face-to-face communication. *Developmental Psychology*, 52: 556–571.

On grounded (context-bound) reasoning: Littleton, K. and Mercer, N. (2018). *Interthinking: Putting Talk to Work*. London: Routledge. Bonnardel, N., Wojtczuk, A., Gilles, P.-Y., and Mazon, S. (2018). The creative process in design. In Lubart, T. (ed.), *The Creative Process*. London: Palgrave. See also various works from the Centre for Real World Learning, especially *Thinking Like an Engineer* in conjunction with the Royal Academy of Engineering, at: www.winchester.ac.uk/realworldlearning. Shteynberg, G., Hirsch, J. B., Bentley, R. A., and Garthoff, J., *et al.* (2020). Shared worlds and shared minds: a theory of collective learning and a psychology of common knowledge. *Psychological Review*. DOI: 10.1037/rev0000200.

For recent relational/constructivist ideas in language theory: Jackendoff, R. and Audring, J. (2020). Relational morphology: a cousin of construction grammar. *Frontiers in Psychology*, 11: 2241. DOI: 10.3389/fpsyg.2020.02241.

For assumptions underlying cognitive theories: Richardson, K. (2020). *Models of Cognitive Development*. London: Routledge.

Chapter 8

For papers on hunter-gatherers: Panter-Brick, C., Layton, R. H. and Rowley-Conwy, P. (eds) (2001). *Hunter-Gatherers: An Interdisciplinary Perspectives*. Cambridge: Cambridge University Press.

On the origins of social class structures: Marrison, R. (2020). Ancient Mesopotamia social classes: www.historyten.com/mesopotamia/ancient-mesopotamia-social-classes.

For concepts of entitlement: Edmiston, D. (2017). How the other half live: poor and rich citizenship in austere welfare regimes. *Social Policy & Society*, 16: 315–325.

Discussion of effects of class structure on self-concept mediating school preparedness (including results from China): Li, S., Xu, Q., and Xia, R. (2020). Relationship between SES and academic achievement. *Frontiers in Psychology*. DOI: 10.3389/fpsyg.2019.02513

On health and well-being related to social class: Jackson, B., Richman, L. S., LaBelle, O., *et al.* (2015). Experimental evidence that low social status is most toxic to well-being when internalized. *Self and Identity*, 14:2, 157–172. See also Loi. M., Del Savio, L., and Stupka, E. (2013). Social epigenetics and equality of opportunity. *Public Health Ethics*, 6: 142–153. For a succinct summary of background 'factors' associated with educational outcomes, see the Equality Trust: www.equalitytrust.org.uk.

For critical views of the environment: Mayes, L. C. and Lewis, M. (2012). *The Cambridge Handbook of Environment in Human Development*. Cambridge: Cambridge University Press.

For systemic consequences of extreme environments experienced during development: Nugent, B. and McCarthy, M. M. (2015). Epigenetic influences on the developing brain: effects of hormones and nutrition. *Advances in Genomics and Genetics*, 5: 215–225. See also the study by Mackes, N. K., Golm, D., Sarkar, S., *et al.* (2020). Early childhood deprivation is associated with alterations in adult brain structure despite subsequent environmental enrichment. *Proceedings of the National Academy of Sciences USA*, 117: 641–649.

For a critical review of the concept of giftedness: Freeman, J. (2006), Giftedness in the long term. *Journal for the Education of the Gifted*, 29: 384–403. For a wider review: Myers, T., Carey, E., and Szücs, D. (2017). Cognitive and neural correlates of mathematical giftedness in adults and children: a review. *Frontiers in Psychology*, 8: 1646. DOI: 10.3389/fpsyg.2017.01646. For a different view: Kaufman, S. B. (2017). *Ungifted: Intelligence Redefined*. New York: Basic Books.

On giftedness in Einstein: Janssen, M. and Renn, J. (2015). History: Einstein was no lone genius. *Nature*, 527: 298–300.

Scientists on race and genetics: Yudell, M., Roberts, D., DeSalle, R., and Tishkoff, S. (2016). Taking race out of human genetics. *Science*, 351(6273): 564–565. Panofski, A., Dasgupta, K., and Iturriaga, N. (2020). How White nationalists mobilize genetics: from genetic ancestry and human biodiversity to counterscience and metapolitics. *American Journal of Physical Anthropology*. DOI: 10.1002/ajpa.24150.

Chapter 9

Predicting educational performance: Anders, J., Dilnot, C., Macmillan, L., and Wyness, G. (2020). Grade expectations: how well can we predict future grades based on past performance? Centre for Education Policy and Equalising Opportunities, UCL Institute of Education. Richardson, M., Abraham, C., and Bond, R. (2012). Psychological correlates of university students' academic performance: a systematic review and meta-analysis. *Psychological Bulletin*, 138: 353–387.

Predictability of medical school performance: McManus, I., Woolf, K., Dacre, J., *et al.* (2013). The academic backbone: longitudinal continuities in educational achievement from secondary school and medical school to MRCP(UK) and the specialist register in UK medical students and doctors. *BMC Medicine*, 11: 242. DOI: 10.1186/1741-7015-11-242. MacKenzie, R. K., Cleland, J. A., Ayansina, D., *et al.* (2016). Does the UKCAT predict performance on exit from medical school? A national cohort study. *BMJ Open*, 6(10): e011313.

On use of IQ-type tests to boost predictability: Benton, T. and Lin, Y. (2011). *Investigating the Relationship Between A Level Results and Prior Attainment at GCSE*. Slough: National Foundation for Educational Research.

Poor predictability of IQ and school attainments for later achievement: Imlach, A.-R., Ward, D. D., Stuart, K. E., *et al.* (2017). Age is no barrier: predictors of academic success in older learners. *Science of Learning*, 2: 13. DOI:10.1038/s41539-017-0014-5. For life in the real world: Armstrong, J. S. (2011). Natural learning in higher education. In *Encyclopedia of the Sciences of Learning*. London: Springer.

On hollow meritocracy in education, see Sandel, M. (2020). *The Tyranny of Merit: What's Become of the Common Good?* New York: Allen Lane.

For comments on the Finnish school system: https://pasisahlberg.com.On 'Vygotskian' attempts to change school curricula: Erbil, D. E. (2020). A review of Flipped Classroom and cooperative learning method within the context of Vygotsky Theory. *Frontiers in Psychology*. DOI: 10.3389/fpsyg.2020.01157.

An OECD-sponsored review: Kautz, T., Heckman, J. J., Diris, R., *et al.* (2015). Fostering and measuring skills: improving cognitive and non-cognitive skills to promote lifetime success. National Bureau of Economic Research Working Paper 20749.

On concepts of environment: Ball, N., Mercado, E., and Orduña, I. (2019). Enriched environments as a potential treatment for developmental disorders: a critical assessment. *Frontiers in Psychology*. DOI: 10.3389/fpsyg.2019.00466.

On compensatory education: Melhuish, E., Belsky, J., and Barnes, J. (2015). Sure Start and its evaluation in England. In Tremblay, R. E., Boivin, M., and Peters, R. (eds), *Encyclopedia on Early Childhood Development*: www.child-encyclopedia.com/integrated-early-childhood-development-services/according-experts/sure-start-and-its-evaluation.

Critique of neuroscience proposals for education: Bowers, J. S. (2016). The practical and principled problems with educational neuroscience. *Psychological Review*. DOI: 10.1037/rev0000025.

On cognitive enhancement programmes: Farah, M. J. (2015). The unknowns of cognitive enhancement. *Science*, 350: 379–380.

On AI promises: Fjelland, R. (2020). Why general artificial intelligence will not be realized. *Humanities and Social Sciences Communications*, 7: 10. DOI: 10.1057/s41599-020-0494-4. Beede, E., Baylor, E. E., Hersch, F., *et al.* (2020). A human-centered evaluation of a deep learning system deployed in clinics for the detection of diabetic retinopathy. In *CHI '20: Proceedings of the 2020 CHI Conference on Human Factors in Computing Systems*. DOI: 10.1145/3313831.3376718.

Index

Locators in *italic* refer to figures